MASTERING VITALITY

7 Simple & Sustainable Steps To

Lose Weight, Live Pain-Free,

Energize Your Life

& Gain Power

NOW!

Linell King, M.D.

MASTERING VITALITY

7 <u>Simple</u> & <u>Sustainable</u> Steps To

Lose Weight, Live Pain-Free,

Energize Your Life

& Gain Power

NOW!

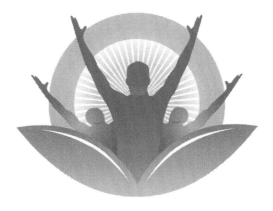

LINELL KING, M.D.

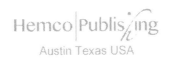

Hemco | Publishing
Austin Texas USA

DISCLAIMER

Requests for permission should be addressed to:
Wellness Consultants of Naples,
Attn: Rights and Permissions Department
5275 Collier Blvd #201 PMB #226
Naples, FL 34119

FIRST EDITION

Achieve Ultimate Vitality is a registered trademark of Wellness Consultants of Naples, LLC a Linell King, MD company.

Cover Design, Format, and Layout by Hemco Publishing

Managing Editor: Susan Hemme

Cover Photo by Anna Nguyen

ISBN- 978-1494433192

DEDICATION

Because of you, Pop, I have ventured upon this journey and have become
the man I am today. May your spirit forever reside not only in me,
but also in everyone who is touched by this book.

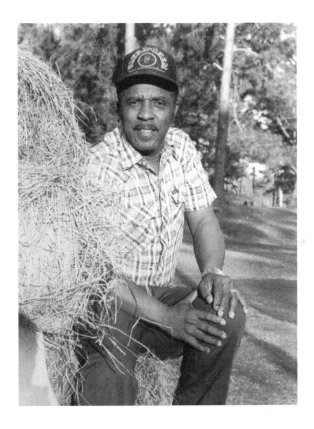

Richard Clinton King
November 11, 1931 - November 15, 1999

Contents

MASTERING VITALITY

7 Simple & Sustainable Steps To

Lose Weight, Live Pain-Free,

Energize Your Life

& Gain Power

NOW!

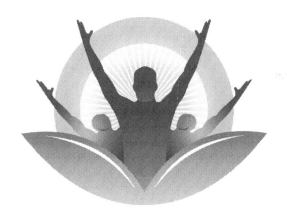

Linell King, M.D.

Preface

By Linell King, M.D.

Hello. My name is Linell King, and I honor you for taking this time to improve your health. For you to pick up a book like this tells me you are among the elite few who strive to be the best, achieve high, fail fast, and are willing to do whatever it takes to live your life to it's fullest. However, like most of us, you have challenges that are affecting your health, whether it is diet, lack of weight control, too many medications, battling sleep disorder, or any other challenge. You know you have the capability to do more, be more, have more, and give more, but you might be uncertain as to what is holding you back. Am I right? Well, I commend you. You are not alone on this journey for excellence. Every one of us has something to overcome, and that is why I wrote this book. I am here for you as a doctor, a mentor and a friend. My hope is to give you the tools you need to take your health and wellness to the next level. You know what I'm talking about; that level in which you know in your soul you were born to live.

Before we get into the **7 Simple & Sustainable Steps to Mastering Vitality**, let me further introduce myself to you. At the young age of six, I decided I wanted to be a doctor. It was not because I was health conscious in any way at that time. I started out wanting to be a plumber, just like my dad. However, when I went to work with him, I found out how hard his job was and I knew that manual labor was not for me. What I did enjoy was going to my pediatrician. He was a fun person who truly cared about me… he even gave me an apple every time I went to see him! Because of that, and the fact that doing his job looked easier than what my dad did every day, I decided to follow in his footsteps. Then, while I was in college, I actually worked with a pediatrician. But all I did was hold kids down while they got their shots! Needless to say, I did not want to be a pediatrician anymore, although, I did still want to be a doctor.

In the medical field, you have to make a decision between two broad fields, either general medicine or a specialty (i.e. surgery). I really enjoyed surgery, but I wanted to help people without necessarily just cutting out the problem. Because of the broad range of options available, I chose internal medicine. This allows me to do what I enjoy as well as focus on each person as a whole. Being a doctor certainly empowers me to help people who are sick, but it was because of my dad that it became my mission in life to help people like you prevent getting sick in the first place.

You see, my dad was, and always will be my hero. He is in the core of who I am today. He was all about the values of accomplishment, doing the work and caring for his family. His story is more of a "rags to accomplishment" story than it is a story of riches, although he did provide a great life for our family including fun vacations, cars, motorcycle, RV, and a boat as well as renovating our Los Angeles home. He worked multiple jobs and became a highly sought-after plumber, even being hired by some amazing celebrities such as Ray Charles. Pop was successful in his own right. He had such great skills, was well respected by celebrities, took care of the people he worked for, and also had a genuine care for our family. In fact, he cared so much that when he realized the city life was risky for a young black male such as myself, he risked everything and moved us to rural Alabama. Although we were living a cleaner, safer lifestyle, the culture in that area of Alabama did not support the plumber trade. People paid my father with favors and chickens (none of which we could spend). So he supported us by working at a correctional facility then later he applied for a job with the Evergreen Housing Authority. This was not just any job, it was for the position of Director! What made this amazing was that my father never finished high school. He was the youngest of thirteen children and had to help support the family. It was later that he received his GED and took up plumbing as a trade. You can imagine that aiming for the director position for the housing authority was a stretch, to say the least! I was around 12 years old at the time and vividly remember when he got the job. He came home so ecstatic, as if he had just won the lottery! I never saw Pop so animated. I was too young to know what he had just accomplished, but I knew it was something amazing.

He instilled in me the belief that I could do anything I set my mind to. He never said as much, but simply lived this value and showed me by example. Do the work, accomplish your best, and care about people.

With his new job, Pop reinvented the meaning of low-income housing in our city. He renovated the projects and built a completely new development. His goal was to create the nicest possible development in town. He refused to allow anyone to refer to them as "the projects" and as a result, he accomplished that goal. He was a truly enterprising person. While managing this job, my dad also purchased a country convenience store, which he and my mom both ran.

We lived on a farm with our own livestock and grew our own vegetables and crops. It was great living with clean air and good old-fashioned southern cooking made with home grown and raised food. Pop loved to barbeque, and all of our meals were centered on meat. Fried chicken, steak, pork, you name it. At the time, I thought the southern diet was a good diet. It wasn't your typical processed fast foods that many people eat in the city. I thought that we were living a healthy lifestyle. What did I know? It was how we were raised.

My dad was built like Popeye. I never dreamed he would ever get sick. In my eyes, he was healthy. He worked hard, rarely had a drink, and didn't smoke. I'd never seen him cry or break down. We were very tight. He was the best man in my wedding and my best friend in life. Pop supported every crazy aspiration of mine, no matter how ludicrous it sounded, including me becoming a doctor.

During my residency at The Johns Hopkins University School of Medicine, my Mom called to say that Pop was having some indigestion and had gone to the doctor. They were told he had a mass on his pancreas. This news hit me like a ton of bricks.

Feeling the blood fall from my face I asked, "Mom, are you sure?" I could hear the concern in her voice as she said, "Yes I... think so."

I instantly knew what "mass on his pancreas" translates into...Cancer. Moreover, pancreatic cancer, at the time of diagnosis, yields a form of death sentence. What had just happened was that my mom told me that my hero, my superman, my rock, *my dad, her husband...* would no longer be alive in four months.

"Mom, are you sure it's not the prostate or something like that?"

"No son, they said the pancreas."

I instantly flew home to explain to my parents that Pop might not see another Christmas. To this date, it has been the hardest thing I have ever had to do. My dad said he wanted to fight, so we got the best surgeon and the best oncologist (physician who deals with cancer) in Alabama. He went through an extremely invasive and painful procedure and spent an entire month in the hospital. Of course, I took a leave of absence from residency to be by my parents' side. My dad spent 25% of his expected survival time in the hospital recovering from this horrendous procedure. After surgery, the prognosis was the same. We were devastated.

The next month Pop spent his time at home learning to walk and eat again. He decided against chemo but still wanted to fight. I had learned of an optimal wellness clinic in San Diego and decided to take him there. Sadly, my mom had to stay behind and run the store. Pop and I had scheduled to spend two weeks at the wellness center, but had to return home early because of fluid build-up in his lungs.

Here is the astounding part of the story: During our time at the wellness clinic, I learned more about health and wellness than in all four years of medical school! Medical school taught me about disease, not health. This wellness center taught me about health. Pop and I were shocked at all the information about living foods, nutrition, the digestive system, wheat grass, etc.

I remember he looked at me with his sunken eyes and said, "If only I had known about this sooner."

I replied, "Me too, Pop. Me too."

Two months later during the week of Thanksgiving, my hero died.

After we laid my dad to rest, I let grieving have its way with me and found myself neglecting my own health. You wouldn't think it, right? I just did not want to deal with his death (nor did I have the skills that I have now to take care of myself holistically). I found myself in a place where I was about 25 pounds overweight, sluggish, experiencing back pain, had a lot of inflammation in my joints, and was feeling lethargic and unfulfilled. I did not consciously know it at the time, but much of what I was feeling was also a result of ignoring my mission. I focused on work. For about ten years, I tried dieting to lose the weight, but then I would gain it right back (you know that annoying Yo-Yo dieting cycle). I had all of the right knowledge, but I was subconsciously blocking myself from doing what I knew I needed to do. Finally, I got fed up and made the commitment to change my life, once and for all.

It all came together for me when I combined everything I had learned from medical school, the wellness center, other learning channels, and a one-year world tour with life mastery expert, Tony Robbins. I literally educated and reprogrammed myself on every level possible. As a result, not only did I easily lose the weight and reverse the pain and inflammation, but also I felt highly energetic and fully alive! I now *sustain* being truly healthy, inside and out. Good-bye Yo-Yo!!

If it worked for me, it will work for everybody, right? But how can you achieve these results without having to invest years of your life (and tons of money) going as deep into the learning process as I did? Well, I decided to analyze that. I took a look at what I was doing differently now on a daily basis (physically, mentally, emotionally and spiritually) and discovered a clear and concise pattern of seven different things. These seven things, which I developed into the 7 Steps in this book, are literally the key to sustainable success.

I decided to try this with my clients. (Note that I identified them as clients because when I refer patients, I am referring to those who are sick and quite possibly in the hospital. Therefore when I see people outside of the hospital they are not patients, they are clients). I wanted to make sure that this was something I could duplicate so that when people like you need help with things (i.e. weight loss, chronic illness, medication reduction or elimination, etc.), I could successfully guide you and treat your life as a whole.

Well, it worked. These same 7 Steps were just as effective for my clients without them having to go through the trials and tribulations I went through in order to bring this information to you. I simply serve as the bridge between traditional board-certified internal medicine physicians and alternative holistic wellness-minded naturopathic practitioners. In addition, the 7 Steps are the stepping-stones on your pathway to true health and vitality.

So, there you have it, the story about what motivated me to develop the **7 Simple & Sustainable Steps to Mastering Vitality** and the magnificent man behind it all who inspired me. I could never describe how difficult it was to lose my dad. Nevertheless, I find peace in knowing that his life mattered, not only because of his accomplishments and the positive impact he had on those around him, but also in the legacy he instilled in me to care for others and make a difference in the world. It was through him that my mission to help you live in your best health came to light. Whatever it takes, I am here to serve you… one step at a time.

Linell King, M.D.

Introduction

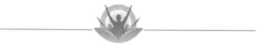

MASTERING VITALITY

"Mastering Vitality means gaining control of your own health so that you can maximize your energy and live a stronger, more extraordinary life." - **Linell King, M.D.**

Have you (or someone you know) ever had cancer? Have you (or someone you know) ever lost someone you loved to a heart attack? Do you know anybody who has been limited, debilitated, or diagnosed with diabetes? How about obesity or problems with controlling your weight? I could go on asking you questions like these, and unfortunately, statistics dictate you will answer "Yes" more times than "No". Currently, one out of every four Americans dies of heart disease. Over 1.6 million men, women and children have some form of cancer, and more than 25.8 million of our family, friends and neighbors are being diagnosed with a prevalence of diabetes in the U.S. That means 100% of those people are sick! Tragically, they are sick as a direct result of poor choices in diet and lifestyle that will lead to weight gain, illnesses, diseases, and ultimately, loss of life. Fortunately, because this is result of choice, this can change.

Here's another question for you. Did you know that on average, illnesses and diseases are approximately 40% advanced in your body before you ever experience your first symptom? Take a moment to think about what I just said, *forty percent.* This why most people think they are healthy, when in fact, they are not! For example, let's take diabetes (known as the silent killer) – symptoms are increased hunger, thirst, and/or urination, which do not show up until the disease is well advancing in your body. So, let me ask you, how long will it take for you to notice this as a state of crisis in your body before you take action to correct it? Is it possible that this disease is already manifesting itself in your body this very moment? Is it possible?

Heart Disease, Cancer, and Diabetes Are All Preventable Killers!

That's right, preventable. If these illnesses are preventable, then this means that *you* have control over the direction and destiny of your own health. ***You control your health***.

Of course, worrying about illness and disease is not the only thing that should motivate you to make wiser choices. What about how the state of your health (and weight) is affecting your life right now? How is this interfering with your family, your career, your performance, or your social life? What is it doing to your self-esteem or the way you think of how others view you?

There is a wealth of information and data available that backs up what I give you here in **7 Simple & Sustainable Steps to Mastering Vitality.** I encourage you to get all the knowledge you need and find what works for you. It is more important than ever to educate yourself on your *own* body rather than thinking that the answer is somewhere outside of you; this book will help you with that education as well as implementing into your own life.

The best way for you to read this book is to go through it with an open mind. I invite you to enjoy the information and stories while focusing on how they would apply to you and your situation. This is an opportunity for you to get clear on what you want for yourself, discover what is blocking you and see what you can do to move forward. You will read about Bob, a 62-year old successful entrepreneur who (before implementing the 7 Steps) was at high risk for the killers mentioned above. You will also learn how he overcame challenges to lose over 100 lbs. in order to reclaim his life, improve the sexual relationship with his wife and save his marriage! You will also read about David, who at a much younger age of 45 used the 7 Steps to conquer poor eating habits due to ethnic and cultural issues. I will tell you about Mary (ironically, Bob's ex-wife) and others who started out like you (and me, for that matter) unaware of the risks and consequences of what our society deems to be normal, and how you can begin now to turn that around.

Your *Mastering Vitality* Simple Plan. Each chapter is designed to build on previous chapters and give you what you need to improve your life. At the end of each chapter, commit to doing at least ONE ACTION item that you can start today, and then turn to Chapter 8 and write that down in the area provided for you (or write in your journal, on note sheet in your smart phone, or on any piece of paper – whatever works for you). This is the foundation for making your simple plan and creating the life that you deserve.

Your Prescription for Mastering Vitality. By the end of this book, my hope is that you will have an understanding of the **7 Simple & Sustainable Steps to Mastering Vitality** as well as a completed written Simple Plan. You will find your Prescription for Mastering Vitality in the Summary along with options for how you can get your prescription filled.

Acknowledgements

I have worked hard to put this information together for you and I am very humble to be in a place to offer you this book. This entire process has been amazing, from writing this book, launching my radio show and providing coaching, mentoring and VIP programs to speaking and putting on live events. You being in your best health is what motivates me to do what I do. I admit it has not been easy, however I have been most fortunate to have the tremendous support of like-minded people who have helped me to accomplish my physical, personal and professional goals.

I would like to thank my Mom, Shirley King for her ever-present love and undying support, which have helped me to continue to push forward no matter what challenges I was faced with.

I thank my editor and friend, Susan Hemme for helping me to make this book happen.

I especially give thanks to my Anthony Robbins Platinum Partners, my accountability and mastermind groups, business partners and dear friends, all of who have helped to keep me on the right path.

Most importantly, I give special thanks to all of you reading this book. I appreciate you for taking the time to hear what I have to say. I know your lives are extremely busy and I want you to know that I do not take that lightly. So, without further ado, here are the **7 Simple & Sustainable Steps to Mastering Vitality** for you to enjoy in good health!

Chapter 1

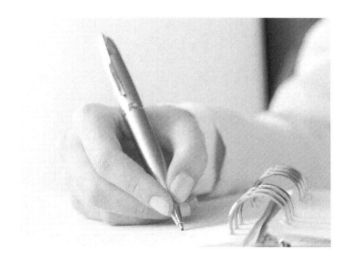

CLARITY

STEP 1 of 7 Steps to Mastering Vitality

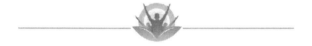

Okay, so you are ready to make lasting change in your life. Sounds simple, right? You would think so, but if it were that easy, everybody would just do it and there wouldn't be books like this. Most people just don't know what to do or in what order in which to do it. Once you have that figured out, the rest is easy, but you will never sustain what you really want for yourself unless you have absolute clarity as to where you are now and where it is you want to go.

Absolute clarity means getting clear in *all* areas of your life. That means knowing what you want, where you want to be, and what it takes for you to get there. Before this can be accomplished, you must also be clear about your environment, your surroundings, and the body in which you live.

Awareness of Your Environment

We live in a culture that is fast-paced and money-driven. Our food supply in the last 30 years has drastically changed to keep up with that demand, and the majority of foods available to you today are no longer nearly as good as they were when you were growing up. Anything that is manufactured, packaged, or served to you through a drive-up window is over-processed in a way that not only destroys the nutritional values and quality of the food, but also contains chemicals and toxins that are sure to create havoc to your health.

Educating yourself on the foods you eat, the air you breathe and the world in which you live is important. Information is power, however only if you then take action on that information. I suggest you reach out to every resource available to you and learn everything you possibly can about the overall environment and how it affects your health.

Get Clear on Your Surroundings

Home is where the heart is, as well as where your health begins. I understand the challenges that your surroundings can have on you personally as I too have had to deal with these issues in my own life. Nevertheless, that does not mean that you have to be subjected to a way of life that does not serve you. The way for you to gain control is to first get clear on what is both supporting you as well as challenging you in attaining your goals. Amplify that which supports you and tweak the rest.

This is what I suggest to help you get clear: Take a look around and list everything that you appreciate. Also, list everything that you feel is holding you back. What are your surroundings like? Is it clean and organized or unclean and messy? Are the people you hang out with progressive, positive, and healthy or reactionary, negative and tired? Is your home filled with items that are energizing such as music, clean foods and things that stimulate activity, or is it filled with junk foods and televisions that are constantly blaring? What is your bedroom like? What are your work surroundings? How about your car?

Write your answers to these questions so that you have a list of things to be grateful for as well as a list of things to improve. This type of clarity gives you a starting point for your focus of change.

Listen to Your Body!

Another step in gaining clarity is to maximize the resources that you have within you. As a leader, you empower your team by listening to those in the trenches and then making the appropriate corrections, right? Well, as a Master of Vitality and the leader of your own destiny, the smartest thing you can do is listen to your body.

We have been blessed, and cursed, with our power to think. Because of these very powerful brains, we have unfortunately suppressed the innate intelligence of our bodies. To illustrate this point, let me give you an example. When you lose one faculty (such as sight, smell, hearing, taste, or touch) another sense becomes stronger. E.g. if you lose your eyesight, your hearing improves. However, the opposite is true when we rely upon our thinking too much because we then override, *or ignore* our natural senses.

When trying to decide what is right or wrong for your body, I have found the best direction to follow is to mimic nature. Think about it. When you look at the animals, you know that they do not have to go through years of college or medical school to educate themselves about their bodies or what to eat. How do they know what is or is not poisonous or toxic? They know because they innately listen to the natural senses in their bodies. They do not have the level of thought process that we humans do, so their sense of being in tuned with their bodies is much higher than ours. When it comes to pain or problems, unlike the animals, we think the smart thing to do is take medications.

Medications are NOT the cure. They just cover up the symptoms. Symptoms are our body's way of telling us to change our actions. We have become the reactionary product of highly effective marketing and powerful, money-driven drug industries. There is a pill for everything. I am not saying that medications are not needed. Medications can be life-saving when administered at the appropriate times, but they also are overused and abused. Our society has been conditioned in a way that our brains tell us if we eat something that causes heartburn then that means we need to take medicine. Yet our bodies are really just telling us to stop eating foods that gave us heartburn! It is really that simple!

Symptoms have a purpose. When you eat something that causes harm, your body will send a warning signal. When a baby cries, it is not because they have an attitude, it is because they need something and are trying to get somebody's attention in order to give it to them. So just like the cry of a baby, the pain or discomfort that your body is delivering says, "Hey, something is wrong! Can you please correct it?"

Food allergies, hormonal imbalances, loss of weight control, and all symptoms of pain and discomfort are simply your body's way of communicating to you. Being clear on this gives you the control you need to take action and set goals, not only to correct the problems you have, but also to prevent them in the first place.

SET CLEAR AND CONCISE GOALS

Have you tried to drop a few pounds only to gain it all back again? Believe me, this is quite common. Over and over again, I hear clients say that they want to lose weight, yet they are unclear about what that really means. For example, a typical conversation goes like this:

"I want to lose weight."

"How much weight do you want to lose?"

"Well, I don't know, 20 or 30 pounds."

"That's a big difference, 20 or 30 pounds. Why do you want to lose weight?"

"Oh, I just know I need to."

Saying you want to lose weight without clarity is like saying you want to go west without knowing if you'll end up in California or Timbuktu. You must be able to clearly see the picture, and that comes in three parts: knowing where you are, knowing where you want to be, and then putting yourself there.

Know Where You Are

In order for you to know where you are, you must first take 100% responsibility for being there! Your life, your health, and every aspect of the way you live is a result of every thought and every choice you have made up until this very moment. The way you think creates your reality for yourself. How you think and what you choose to do is based upon where you put your focus.

Take Mary for instance. She would stand on her scale in front of a full-length mirror, naked, and curse everything she did not like about her body. She had gained nearly 25 lbs. since her divorce from Bob, and all she saw, in her words, was "a big fat ass, blubbery thighs and saggy boobs." Can you imagine the mental state she was putting herself in?

Mary wanted to date and fall in love again, yet she blamed the condition of her body as the reason for not being able to attract men. She complained about lack of energy and feeling bad emotionally. In her mind, she had tried everything to lose weight and nothing worked. This was not true. What Mary didn't understand was that by focusing on what was wrong with her body, she was creating a disempowering belief system that led to her own unhappiness. She then subconsciously turned to comfort food to make herself feel better, when in fact it was one of the very things that was making her feel worse! Mary saw herself as a victim of circumstance, yet *she* was the one allowing her own thoughts to interfere with what she really wanted for herself. Therefore, *she* was the one who was in control.

The beauty of taking responsibility for what is wrong with your life is that you also get to take credit for all that is good; Therein lies your power. When I work with clients like Mary, one of the first things I do is help you to identify where you might be sabotaging yourself. You will then be able to shift your focus towards areas of your life that are working to your benefit. Mary learned to shift her focus away from "being" fat to giving herself credit for stepping up and making the change. Rather than feeding herself comfort foods in order to feel better emotionally, she focused on feeding herself live foods so that she could look and feel better in the long run. And instead of standing on her scale, naked and cursing, she used that time to smile in the mirror, congratulate herself and be grateful for what was right. By taking full responsibility and shifting her focus, Mary began to take control of her life and feel better about what she could do with it.

She was then ready, willing, and able to make a simple plan for herself that would be long lasting rather than just another fad diet.

Know Where You Want to Be

In order to make a plan that will work, you have to know where you want to end up and what you want it to look like when you get there. You may know that you want to lose 20 pounds of excess body fat, but you need to be crystal-clear on what that will mean to you. Losing 20 pounds of fat from liposuction surgery is certainly going to give you a different result than loosing 20 pounds of fat by making lifestyle changes! One goal is to lose weight; the other is to achieve your ideal weight and thrive.

Your overall health, and wellness is more than just your physical body. Along with your physical vitality, there is your mental, emotional, spiritual, sexual, environmental, financial vitalities, etc. As you set your goals, get clear on everything that surrounds you. It is important to know as a whole, what you want for your holistic vitality.

Start by defining what vitality means for you, what that translates into, and how it applies to your entire life. Take a moment and make a list of everything you want. What do you want for yourself? What do you want to feel like? Who do you want in your life? What do you want those relationships to be like? Where do you want to live? Where do you want to work? How do you want to spend your free time? How do you want to connect spiritually? Who do you want to become? What do you want to be known for? What legacy do you want to leave?

Compare your findings to where you are currently in life. By getting clear on where you are and where you want to be, you are able to see the gap in between. For example, when Bob started this process, he wanted to lose weight and guessed he should be aiming it to be around 50 pounds. That was it. But once he got clear that he wanted to look and feel like he did just after college so that he could do more, increase his business, live longer, be a better father, have a better sexual relationship with his wife and improve his marriage, he then clearly saw the gap between where he was and what it was going to take for him to get there. In actuality, Bob needed to lose over 100 pounds *and* he needed to minimize his risk for diseases, maximize his energy, get his hormones tested and certainly increase his vitality!

Put Yourself There

The 2006 movie, ***The Secret***, popularized the idea of being able to get everything you want by simply believing, feeling good, thinking positively, and visualizing yourself already having that which you wish to obtain. This principal, known as "The Law of Attraction," was endorsed by many successful celebrities such as Oprah Winfrey, Will Smith and Jim Carrey to name a few. While the concept of visualizing yourself already being where you want to be is good, by itself it is not enough to gain the clarity you need in order to make something happen. You need to also evoke "The Law of Action". In other words, don't just think and feel yourself there… PUT yourself there. Let me explain.

After my dad died, there were about ten years when I went through the motions of taking care of myself, but I was not fully applying the principals that I am sharing with you now. If you recall in the story that I told in the Preface, I gained about 25 pounds accompanied by assorted health issues (and being a doctor, I should have known better)! I knew where I was… I was overweight and feeling bad. I knew what I wanted for myself... I wanted to be healthy and vibrant. I imagined myself thinner, but my thoughts were inconsistent with my actions. I would lose weight, gain it back, lose weight, and gain it back. I would certainly *visualize* myself healthy, but it wasn't until I made the decision to *be* healthy and *do* whatever it took to actually put myself there that I would finally get the results. I had to take action – relentless, fully-committed, no-nonsense ACTION!

Do not get me wrong. I am a total fan of visualization. It is important, as well as highly effective, to visualize yourself being in the state of health you want to be. I believe in creating vision boards for yourself where you can post words and pictures of things you want to create in your life. The fine line is, rather than just imagining yourself healthy, also *take immediate action to be healthy.* This gives you momentum, and in each moment, you will gain more and more clarity that your goal is being realized.

Starting right now, you can put yourself in a state of being healthy by thinking, feeling, acting and *doing* healthy in every moment of your life going forward. When Mary stood on her scale cursing, she was *doing* the actions of a fat person who only wished to lose weight. When she praised herself in the mirror and showed gratitude for all that was right in her life, she was able to instantly put herself in the state she wanted to be by *doing* the actions of a happy, healthy person. It is that simple. *Put yourself there*: think the right thoughts, do the right actions and your body will follow.

REVIEW: CLARITY

1. Get clear in every aspect of your life. Decide specifically on the goals that you desire and write them down.
2. Be aware of your environment and surroundings; make a list of what you like and do not like.
3. Listen to your body! Symptoms are your body's way of asking for help.
4. Know where you *really* are and take 100% responsibility for being there.
5. Know where you want to be and be very clear on the details

of what that looks like.

6. Put yourself there by visualizing and taking immediate action now to make it happen.

Before you move on to the next level, answer the following questions:

1. What was the MOST VALUABLE THING that you gained from this chapter?*
2. What is the ONE THING that you can put into action TODAY?*

* Turn to **Chapter 8: Mastering Vitality Simple Plan** and write your answers in the area provided for you (or write in your journal, on note sheet in your smart phone or any piece of paper – whatever works for you). This is the foundation for building your simple plan.

NOTE: *It is __IMPORTANT__ that you __TAKE ACTION__ and __GET SUPPORT__. Connect immediately with someone like-minded such as an accountability partner, health coach, or professional mentor. **This is key to your success.** For additional resources, support and a **SPECIAL GIFT** from **Dr. King**, please visit MasteringVitalityNow.com*

Chapter 2

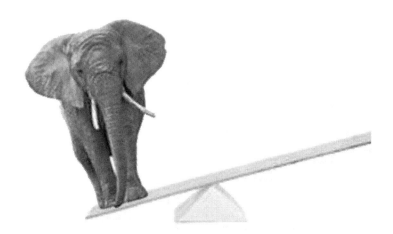

LEVERAGE

STEP 2 of 7 Steps to Mastering Vitality

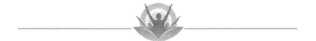

Taking consistent, proactive action is a common thread you will see throughout the **7 Simple & Sustainable Steps to Mastering Vitality**. It is vital to your success. Yet many people tend to fail at following through with things they have started. Why is that? The answer is, leverage. As human beings, we are creatures who naturally want to be comfortable. We avoid pain and seek pleasure. We desire instant gratification and have a tendency to give it to ourselves without considering the consequences.

Subsequently, in order to take *and maintain* the action necessary to make change, we must get leverage on ourselves in a way that is stronger than our desire to feel comfortable.

Basically, leverage is using something to maximize your advantage over something else. Just as you would use mechanical leverage to move an object physically, you can use emotional leverage to motivate yourself to take action. For example, if someone tells you they will give you a million dollars if you can lift an elephant, and they will shoot you in the head if you don't, chances are you will do whatever it takes to lift up that elephant! That person has just used emotional leverage on you, and you will need to use mechanical leverage to get the job done.

GAINING EMOTIONAL LEVERAGE

When you look at how a seesaw works, there is a long, rigid board that hinges on a point in the center called a fulcrum. The closer the fulcrum is to the object you want to lift, the easier it becomes to lift that object. So, as that crazy person stands there with a million dollars and a gun, all you have to do is get a strong enough seesaw with the fulcrum in the right place and then you can lift up that silly elephant. Most people would not want to bother doing this, however, if the *emotional* leverage were strong enough, they would be willing to do so.

To gain emotional leverage on yourself, imagine the object as your goal and the fulcrum as your reason for obtaining that goal. The closer you put that fulcrum to your goal, or the more important you make your reason for reaching it, the more likely you are to be consistent in the action you take in order to make that goal happen. As your doctor and health mentor, I would tell you that maintaining a healthy lifestyle in order to avoid obesity, illnesses and diseases that lead to an early painful death is more than enough reason. However, as your friend and fellow human being, I understand it takes more than that in order to truly gain emotional leverage on yourself.

We are far more inspired to avoid pain than we are to seek pleasure. In other words, you will more than likely lift that elephant to avoid being shot than you would to get the million dollars. Unless you are experiencing illness and disease right now, you might be less likely to take immediate and serious action to correct the state of your health. Here's the rub: Illness and disease IS at your door! Death IS staring you in the face! Diabetes is only one of the silent killers. The first symptom you experience with heart disease is usually angina (chest pain due to lack of blood flow to the heart), stomach upset, a heart attack itself, or no symptoms at all. Right now, your body is filled with cells that have the potential to mutate into cancer cells just waiting for your immune system to break down. In addition, if you are overweight at all, the chance of these diseases taking you out at any minute is highly increased. *Pain is that close!* Unfortunately, most of the very pain you are trying to avoid is cleverly wrapped up in a tasty hamburger, a slab of steak, or a fancy coffee drink. You do not recognize it as pain. Clever marketing has seen to that! Therefore, you will not emotionalize this as an urgent reason to take care of your health.

DETERMINE YOUR "WHY"

Emotional leverage works by using pain and pleasure to move you toward your goals, just as pushing down on the seesaw is used to accomplish the goal of lifting the elephant. If you think of the fulcrum as your reason for doing something, then the more important you make your reason, the more powerful your emotional leverage becomes.

The way to make your reason "Why" more important would be to attach a significant amount of pain and pleasure. When I ask my clients, "*Why* do you want to lose weight?" invariably they do not have a good enough reason. Therefore, we dig deeper until we find it. Once they get in touch with their reason "Why", and make it a big enough reason, they are able to move mountains… or lift an elephant… or whatever they choose to accomplish!

What is Your "Why"?

In many circles, this is also the same as asking you, "What is your Mission?" or "What is your Purpose?" Whatever you choose to call it, the question is, how do you find something that honestly inspires you… something that moves and motivates you? I have discovered the best way is to make a list of what is working or not working in your life as well as list what you want your life to be like in your future.

Discover Your "Why" by Creating Your "Why" List. Take out a piece of paper and draw a line vertically down the middle. On the left side, list of all the ways your current lifestyle has negatively affected your life. Think of all of the things you have not done, all of the places you have not gone, all of the people you have not seen and all of the clothes that you have not worn as a result. What beautiful clothes did you see on someone else that you wished you could wear? How many times have you shrunk into the background? Who haven't you approached at an event or party? What sporting or holiday event did you pass on to avoid embarrassment? When was the last time you adjusted yourself or removed yourself socially because of your weight? What else can you think of? This information completes the left side.

On the right side of the paper, create a list of all of the things you would like to do again, all of the things you would like to try, all of the places you would like to go, and all of the ways mastering vitality would change your life. What relationship would you be in right now if you were healthy, happy and confident? What new adventures would you go on? How proud would you be to attend the next party, fundraiser, wedding, or graduation?

Be sure to go back to your left column and add anything you just thought of that you might have missed, and then continue adding all of the things that you want to do on the right column. Keep doing this until you have exhausted every thought (the good, the bad, and the ugly).

Look at the list on the left. What is it about your life that you want to change? What problems has your lack of fitness caused you? What problems will it cause if you don't change it? What are you missing out on? Have you missed fun games on the beach or activities with children or grandchildren? When you look at yourself in the mirror, what do you see? Do you even *like* what you see?

Now imagine yourself, the new you (from the right column), perfect and sculpted, the way that you want to see yourself. Think about having the energy to play with your children or your grandchildren. Think of being the athlete that you were in high school or college. Think of the person that you used to be when you were active, when you felt vibrant, or when you were your happiest. Is that where you want to be now?

Keep Asking Questions Until You Have Created Leverage on Yourself

Do you wish to live longer? Why? What would you like to do or contribute at certain milestones in your life?

Do you wish to be able to enjoy your golden years rather than living it in pain or discomfort? Describe your ideal self in your golden years.

Would you like to have more energy? What would you do if you had more energy? How would this increased energy affect your life?

Would you want to protect yourself from future medical costs?

Would you like to be able to play and interact with your grandchildren? How about your great grandchildren? Describe the activities and the role you would play with them.

Would you like to increase your productivity and income? How will Mastering Vitality help you achieve this?

Would you like to have the body you have always wanted? Describe your ideal body and fitness level.

Would you like to feel more attractive? Have better sex?

Are there certain clothes that you would like to wear that you feel uncomfortable wearing now? Describe them and how you would feel wearing them.

Would you like to improve your mental health? Think more clearly?

Magnify Your "Why"

Once you have analyzed what your current lifestyle looks like, take full stock of what it will cost if you *don't* change. Multiply that by five years and imagine what your life will become. What will your body look like five years from now? What might be the state of your health? What are you missing out on?

Now multiply that by ten years. What does your body look like now? How much energy do you have? How much pain do you have and what is that doing to your life?

Visualize and Feel the Pain

Now go a step further and think about whom this is going to hurt. Most of us will do more for others than we will do for ourselves. Picture that loved one; it could be a child, someone who depends on you, a spouse, or someone that you dearly care about. If you do not make a change, how will that affect them? How will it harm them? Who will it hurt the most? Focus inward and really feel it. Don't brush over this thought. Visualize it and feel the pain. Stay in the moment until it really hurts. Do whatever it takes to visualize the painful consequences of not following through. How painful is that? What number is it from 1 -10? What will make that pain level an 8? Focus on that for a few minutes. Feel it! What negative consequence would need to happen to make it a 10? If it doesn't cause your eyes to water, then it's not a 10. This is the one time where you want to *feel* the negative consequences.

Now Move to the Positive

Never leave yourself in the negative place. Once you get painful leverage on yourself, move to the positive and start asking empowering questions. Come back to the present. Imagine what it would be like if you *do* change? How will you benefit now? What would change for the better? Will you be happier? Will you have more energy?

Now multiply that by five years. What will you feel like in five years if you *do* make the change? What will your body look like? What will your energy be like? What will it do to your productivity? What will it do to your business? How will it change your relationships?

Then, multiply that again ten years from now. Who will benefit the most from you making those positive changes? How will that affect your loved ones? How will that affect your children? How will that affect your relationships? Your career? Your dreams? Your aspirations? Your life? Really put yourself in that moment and rejoice in how good it feels.

LEVERAGE YOUR ENVIRONMENT

There is so much emotion attached to the way we grew up eating that it is difficult to challenge, especially in the older, more traditional populations. This is very strong in ethnic cultures such as Latin, Hispanic and African-American (especially in the South) where you might not dare to reveal that you are a vegetarian or anything of the sort.

When I go home and visit my friends in Alabama, most of them are about 80 lbs. overweight… actually almost all of them are obese! I feel they look at me as someone who has abandoned where I came from. Most seem to attach living healthy with an unfavorable perception, which makes it a challenge to feel like I can be myself around them.

There are many layers and links attached to culture that holds us back from achieving our goals. Let's talk about how to control your environment while still honoring and feeling respected in the cultures that you choose to thrive.

I grew up in an African-American household where everything surrounded food with traditions that go back generations and deep to the core. If I had gone home and challenged the foods that we ate in our family, I would have been looked upon as challenging my up-bringing. I would hear statements like, "But this is what you grew up on!" The last thing we want is to feel like an outcast or offend anybody, right?

Cultural Identity

One of the things that drive a culture is identity. For example, to this day I am known for the fried turkey that I make every year for Thanksgiving. Even though it isn't something I like to eat anymore, I choose to make it. It is my identity to do so. When I go to a family reunion, it is my cultural belief that I must be on the grill. It is who my father was, who my uncles were, and who I am. It certainly is not who I truly am in my core, but figuratively speaking, it is who I am in the culture that I live. I am known for my skill set on the grill. So in order to control the health of my environment while embracing my cultural identity, I make simple changes to what I put on the grill. Now, I grill all kinds of vegetables! Not only do I still get to experience the connection with everybody, but also everybody still gets to experience me being on the grill. In addition, they get the added benefit of a more nutritious meal! In this case, I changed one simple action without changing what my culture deems as an expected ritual. The result is a healthier outcome; it is about developing the fine art of establishing your own culture by embracing the cultures you choose to be a part of, and then tweaking what you do in order to make it healthier. I do not reject the tradition of barbequing. It is a cultural staple among family reunions, celebrations, holidays, etc. My dad was in front of a grill and I was there by his side. When my son turned five, he was there next to me taking pictures with barbeque tongs in his hands. The difference is, instead of ribs being on the grill, it is now filled with various types of vegetables. Therefore, I am still passing on the tradition. The only thing I have changed is what's on the grill!

Cultural Language

My dad was able to make a profound cultural change in a community when he became the Director of the Evergreen

Housing Authority in the city where we lived. He made a difference by simply changing the language used to describe "The Projects." You see, the surrounding culture was project-minded. Because it was associated with poverty and crime, it was considered a badge of honor to be from a dangerous neighborhood, which as you can imagine led to all sorts of trouble. My dad changed that by redefining what affordable housing was, and as a result, made it the nicest housing complex amongst *all* the housing complexes (not just the affordable ones). He did it by not allowing anyone to call it "The Projects!" It was still low-income housing and it still stood for what it was suppose to stand for. Yet, as a result of simply changing the language, the essence of the complex in that culture shifted to a point of pride, which completely changed the face of it. My dad is a great example of how to make change without attacking the surrounding culture.

Pop knew how powerful lifestyle was, that is why he moved us from Los Angeles to Alabama. If he had known how powerful diet was that would have been another culture that he would have changed within our family. Unfortunately, it was too late for him. Fortunately, it is not too late for you.

Environmental Culture

When I talk about culture, I'm not just referencing ethnic groups. I am also talking about the culture of successful business people (i.e. where clients are wined and dined at steakhouses and party in luxury…things of inactivity). Before you know it, you can go from being the happy businessperson to becoming the fat and happy businessperson, or that fat and happy person gathering with buddies to watch football while drinking beer and eating chips and ribs. The ultimate result: You are heading for a very unhappy ending to your health.

For many of us another struggle would be going into the restaurant environment with family, friends or business associates. You walk in and the smell of fresh baked breads and creamy entrées overwhelm your senses (including your common sense)! Those you came with lose control ordering appetizers, drinks, high-caloric dishes, and of course, dessert. None-the-less, you are in that situation and yet committed to making healthier choices for yourself. What do you do? This was a battle for David who was trying to lose what he referred to as his "cultural weight." Fortunately, David was able to massively gain leverage on the situation by using it as a teach-by-example experience. You see, at the young age of 45 years old, David had experienced a mild heart attack due to eating foods and living a lifestyle just like everyone else in his culture. As a result, his "Why" was very strong, to say the least (change or die). Rather than making everyone else feel bad by lecturing to them or insisting they go to a different restaurant, David simply ordered foods off the menu that were as live and fresh as possible. He would kindly ask the server if the chef could make a few alterations. By setting a non-judgmental example, those he cared about were able to see how they too could make better choices for themselves and still enjoy the company of others.

If you get creative, you will find many ways to gain leverage on yourself. My goal was to remain in good graces with my family culture while still being the master of my own health and well-being. By getting creative, I was able to leverage the grilling situation, tweak the family tradition, and also have a positive impact on the next generations by offering foods that are better for everyone's health. When people see that you are respectful of who they are and what they believe, they are far more willing to respect the same in you. A side effect is that they may even be open to trying it your way!

REVIEW: LEVERAGE

1. Gain emotional leverage by using pain and pleasure to make your reason for reaching your goals important.
2. Determine your "Why" and keep asking questions until you gain emotional leverage on yourself.
3. Magnify your "Why" by feeling the pain if you *don't* change and seeing the pleasure if you do.
4. Get leverage on your environment. Respect your culture and make choices that serve you.
5. Use positive language to evoke positive change.

Before you move on to the next level, answer the following questions:

1. Did you put into ACTION the one thing that you committed to from the previous chapter? *If not, it is time to rock this thing out! Go back and review the chapter, and commit!*
2. What was the MOST VALUABLE THING that you gained from this chapter?*
3. What is the ONE THING that you can put into action TODAY?*

* Turn to **Chapter 8: Mastering Vitality Simple Plan** and write your answers in the area provided for you (or write in your journal, on note sheet in your smart phone or any piece of paper – whatever works for you). This is the foundation for building your simple plan.

NOTE: *It is IMPORTANT that you TAKE ACTION and GET SUPPORT. Connect immediately with someone like-minded such as an accountability partner, health coach, or professional mentor. **This is key to your success.** For additional resources, support and a **SPECIAL GIFT** from **Dr. King**, please visit MasteringVitalityNow.com*

Chapter 3

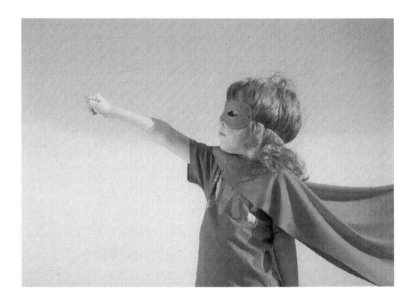

POWER PERSONALITY

STEP 3 of 7 Steps to Mastering Vitality

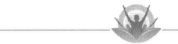

Throughout the world, a wide variety of professionals have expanded upon the understanding and management of different parts of your personality. I have found that when you take control of the parts of your personality that you deem most powerful, you can easily change habits and manage things that seem challenging (such as losing weight). This is highly effective for getting the results you want. In other words, if you want to take control and make things happen, use your Power Personality.

What is a Power Personality?

You are in your power when you have the ability to do, act, or have command over something. Your personality is a combination of the characteristics that form your state of being. If someone is energetic and out-going, you may think he or she has a dynamic personality. If that same person is more sluggish and boring, you might then think they have a dull personality. For most of us, it is normal to shift between several personalities in any given day, depending upon what we are focused on. For example, if you wake up in the morning and focus on how tired you feel, your personality will most likely be dull. However, when you wake up regardless of how you feel, if you focus on being the best that you can be, your personality will be more dynamic. Your Power Personality is when you amplify and utilize the more dynamic part of you that feels unstoppable. How do you do that? You do that through empowering your story and by calling upon the strengths that already live within you.

STORY OF BULLDOZER

When Bob and Mary first met, it was love at first sight. He was a 6' tall, 175 lb. star athlete who was strong, fit, and popular. Mary was a smart little hottie who knew what she wanted out of life. At 5'-5" and 115 lbs., she easily attracted the attention she sought. Shortly after college, the two dynamos were married.

Mary used to refer to Bob as her Bulldozer. "He would just go for it," she recalled. "Nothing could stop him. What Bulldozer wanted, Bulldozer got. That's how he won *me* over!" When Mary talked about what Bob was like back then, she would get a twinkle in her eyes that said far more than this story will ever tell.

Life took over as they settled down and raised a family. Bob's career took off as an investment broker and Mary dedicated her time to being a mom and building her law practice. The more they focused on their businesses, the more successful they became financially. However, their health (and eventually their marriage) suffered as they lost sight of the passions and energies that they had once enjoyed in their youth. Mary slowly gained extra pounds and she fell out of shape. She allowed stress to have it's way with her and turned to fast foods and television for comfort. Her moods easily changed and she became angry over the slightest things. Bob, on the other hand, gained a massive amount of weight as he wined, dined, and entertained his clients. He was always the life of the party, although deep inside he was suffering a lot of emotional pain. The more he tried to please and take care of others, the less he cared for himself. This lifestyle took its toll on Bob and Mary's relationship until, once their kids were grown and after 34 years, they ended the marriage.

As a bachelor again, Bob lost some of the additional weight he had gained. However, after he remarried a younger woman, something shifted in him, and he rapidly put it all back on. The more weight he gained, the less he felt in his power. Then, at over 300 lbs., he could no longer exercise or move as he wanted. He was unable to connect with his clients and found himself passing on a number of business deals. Bob's tests showed that he had signs of diabetes and was at high risk for heart disease. An addition, if that wasn't bad enough… he could no longer have sex with his new wife! His testosterone production had decreased and he was now suffering from erectile dysfunction. Not only had he lost the de

sire, but he had also lost the ability to physically perform!

"If something doesn't change," Bob confided, "she is going to leave me. I don't blame her." There was genuine agony in his eyes. Bob described that every time he started dieting, he would get down to a certain weight but then go back to his old habits again. He felt his new wife distancing from him and knew that he was letting her down. This was a wake up call for Bob. He could see that not only was he heading down the path of fatal disease, but also quite possibly another divorce.

Who was this hurting? Obviously, this was tremendously hurting Bob. When he was at his ideal body weight, he was a star athlete and felt on top of the world. Now he was just the fat guy who knew how to make money; but what good would that be without his health or family? His new wife was fit and beautiful, and he felt that when they hung out people would look at them and wonder why she was with *him*. It was hurting his new wife not to have him there for her emotionally or physically (or not at all). It was also hurting his son, who really looked up to him. He too had started to gain weight and Bob felt like he couldn't talk to him about it because he himself was so big. He saw his son's confidence level dropping in areas of his own life, and Bob knew that he wasn't taking advantage of certain opportunities because of it. Bob's weight was not only hurting him, but it was also hurting his family in an enormous way.

You might be wondering, if Bob could see that this was having an adverse affect on his family, why wasn't he able to do something about it? Well, that's the million-dollar question. There are many reasons that hold people back from successfully making a change. In this case, it was too painful for Bob. He tried not to think about it because when he did, he felt like a failure, got depressed and often ate even more. Bob was in a crisis and more than ever needed to call out his Power Personality – *his life and family depended on it!*

After working though Steps 1 and 2, Bob gained CLARITY and massive emotional LEVERAGE on himself by answering many of the same questions laid out for you. (Anytime you want to gain leverage on yourself, I suggest you go back to Chapter 2 and re-read those questions again.)

Bringing Out the Bulldozer

Following instructions, Bob closed his eyes and remembered what it was like to be the person he used to be when he was at his ideal body weight. He was to feel the way he used to feel, stand the way he used to stand, and breathe the way he used to breathe. As he got into this state, Bob naturally pulled his shoulders back and stood tall and proud as a huge smile came across his face. Then he was asked to give a nickname for that person he was imagining himself to be. Without hesitation he acclaimed, "Bulldozer!" When he was asked to give a nickname for the personality of this person who hangs out around 300 lbs. instead of 175 lbs., he dropped his eyes and shoulders and he sighed, "Bobo."

By simply imagining whether he was Bulldozer or Bobo, Bob realized he had control over which personality he brought forth. *He easily changed his state in an instant by merely focusing on which state he wanted to be in.*

Bobo had served Bob well in many aspects of his life. In some ways, this personality helped him to feel more comfortable and significant. That was the reason why he lived in the Bobo personality for so long. Bobo was also the personality who took care of everyone else and made jokes, even about his own weight. However, Bobo was now tired and could no longer take care of those around him, including Bob. It was time for Bulldozer to take over and start running the show. This translates to retiring that part of you that no longer serves you and bringing forth your personality of strength in order to make the changes that you need. By naming these personalities, they are at your beckon call, giving you full control over them rather than them having control over you.

Bulldozer would not tolerate carrying that extra weight, and he certainly would not allow his new wife to slip away. He was the

Bulldozer for goodness sake! Peak performer! Unstoppable!
Lover man!

As Bulldozer took over, Bobo faded away, the extra pounds began
to melt and the state of Bob's health improved. Bob still wined and
dined his clients, but did so while making wiser choices and
staying connected to his "Why". When it came to dessert, he
would push away from the table, rub his shrinking belly and say,
"No thanks guys, gotta stay in shape for my lady!" Bob paid it
forward by helping his son to find his own Power Personality.
With pride he says, "Like father, like son. Me and my buddy Bob
Cat!"

As for Mary, she recently ran into Bob and could not believe the
transformation. She had seen the changes in their son and heard
they were doing the **7 Simple & Sustainable Steps to Mastering
Vitality**. Bob told her about finding Bulldozer and how he now
lives in that personality and thanked her for giving him that name
years ago. "It really was like talking to the Bulldozer I once
knew," Mary confessed, "and it kind of turned me on!"

Life will never be the same for you after you learn to master this
step! At any given time, especially if you are feeling dull or out of
control, you can master that moment and immediately take charge
by simply calling on (and becoming) your Power Personality.

FINDING YOUR POWER PERSONALITY

Let's break it down. There are four parts to finding your Power
Personality. Please read the following four sections first, then read
over it again and actually DO the exercise. You are about to meet
a very powerful new friend – the real YOU!

Part One: Remember and Relate

Start by remembering a time when you felt in control and on top of your game. Can you remember a time when you felt strong? When did you actually possess the vitality that you are striving for? If nothing comes to mind, whom do you know of who is full of the life and energy that you want for yourself? Can you relate to a personality that you admire? This can be a real person or fictional character, such as an athlete or superhero.

Part Two: Visualize and Become

Close your eyes and visualize the person or character you want to become. Imagine that this is you now. Breathe this energy in. Stand the way that person would stand. Hold your body the same way that person would hold their body. Let your face show that power. *Feel* the POWER! *Become* that POWER! Say something that your Power Personality would say. Now give it a nickname; the *first* name that comes to mind.

Part Three: Retire the Non-Power Personality

Now go back to the non-powerful person or character that you have been living as. You know, the one that made it okay for you to get out of sorts... the one who let you off the hook when it came to achieving your goals. What is that person's name? (Do not use your real name for this personality. By giving it a name of its own, it will help you to disassociate with it.) Let yourself sink into that personality. What does it feel like? Now feel love for that personality and forgive it. Thank it for serving you up until this point. Tell it to rest and that you and your Power Personality will handle things from here on out.

Part Four: Live Your Power Personality!

Go back into your Power Personality again. Now *live* as this new person! Make sure that you step into it fully. Call upon this power to lead the show! Assume the physiology of this person when making decisions. Stand the way this person stands, think the way this person thinks, talk the way this person talks, and use the language that this person uses.

If this is your first time reading this section, now go back, re-read it again, and actually DO the exercise. Do not proceed until you have retired your non-power personality and brought your Power Personality to life! If you have found your Power Personality, CONGRATULATIONS!

It is amazing to see these transformations on stage at my live events. Someone will come up, and depending on what we refer to in their life, they will go into their different personalities. It is amazing to watch the switch happen in front of your eyes. Everyone cheers each other on as they literally see the difference when someone steps into their Power Personality. From that point going forward, we refer to them by their new nickname. This helps to reinforce this personality. I encourage you to invite those around you to call you by your Power Personality name. Additionally, anytime you refer to it yourself, begin with saying, "I am [Power Personality name]" because *this power IS you!*

REVIEW: POWER PERSONALITY

1. Establish CLARITY and LEVERAGE.
2. Identify the part of you that is strong and powerful. Name it.
3. Identify that disempowering part of you. Name it, thank it, and retire it.
4. Now live in your Power Personality!

Before you move on to the next level, answer the following questions:

1. Did you put into ACTION the one thing that you committed to from the previous chapter? *If not, get your Power Personality on! Go back and review the chapter, and commit!*
2. What was the MOST VALUABLE that you gained from this chapter?*
3. What is the name of your POWER PERSONALITY?*
4. What is the ONE THING that you can put into action TODAY?*

* Turn to **Chapter 8: Mastering Vitality Simple Plan** and write your answers in the area provided for you (or write in your journal, on note sheet in your smart phone or any piece of paper – whatever works for you). This is the foundation for building your simple plan.

NOTE: *It is <u>IMPORTANT</u> that you <u>TAKE ACTION</u> and <u>GET SUPPORT</u>. Connect immediately with someone like-minded such as an accountability partner, health coach, or professional mentor. **This is key to your success.** For additional resources, support and a **SPECIAL GIFT** from **Dr. King**, please visit MasteringVitalityNow.com*

Chapter 4

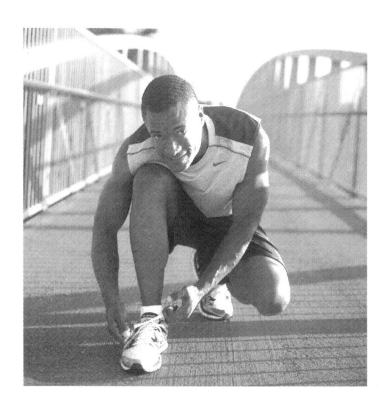

ESSENTIALS

STEP 4 of 7 Steps to Mastering Vitality

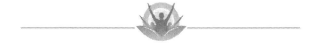

This book is about helping you to master the skills you need in order for you to maximize your health and vitality. Before you can design an optimal plan for yourself, it is important for you to have knowledge of the seven essentials that your body truly needs.

These seven essentials are:

1. Oxygen
2. Water
3. Food
4. Movement
5. Rest
6. Sex
7. Spirituality

This will be the longest chapter for you, but it is critical, so stay with it. In the years I've been practicing medicine, treating patients and working with clients, I have found that in order to achieve the quality of life that you want, these essentials need to be tended to and expressed to their fullest. The more knowledgeable you are on these seven essentials, the faster and easier it will be for you to reach *and sustain* your goals. So let's go through them together. Trust me, you will be glad that you did.

ESSENTIAL #1: OXYGEN

I have never met anyone who can live without breathing. In fact, breathing is one of those things we take for granted. Without thinking about it, we breathe approximately 18 times per minute, over 1,000 times an hour, and nearly 26,000 times a day. Most of us breathe just fine. Yet here's the problem: breathing "just fine" is not optimal. You may get enough oxygen into your blood to support life, but you need to get the optimal amount of oxygen into your blood that will give you an energetic life of vitality.

Poor breathing leads to poor health. Breathing shallow, or holding your breath when you are anxious, restricts oxygen from getting into your blood and vital organs, and causes all sorts of health issues. Purposeful deep breathing works as a quick and easy preventative treatment. It will also help you to improve digestion, develop great posture, and relieve pain.

Our lungs have the capacity to expand more than three times what we use in a normal breath. If you are a woman, my guess is you are especially familiar with the act of pulling in your stomach. Chances are you may do this throughout most of the day. This is not to say men do not pull in their gut from time to time, but women are experts at this. Even though this action can influence core strength, when you flex those abdominal muscles and flatten your abdomen, your diaphragm is pinned against your contracted abdominal muscles, and your breath becomes shallow and ineffectual. This makes it impossible for the diaphragm to properly do its job. Your breathing suffers and therefore, so does the rest of your body. So, let your belly relax and let the air in!

Practice Proper Breathing

To ensure you are properly oxygenating your body, it is advisable to teach yourself to take deep, diaphragmatic breaths so that you are breathing properly. However, the problem with trying to breathe correctly is that our clothes or belts can be too tight, which makes breathing deep into the abdomen uncomfortable. So, if there is anything constricting around your waist, loosen up!

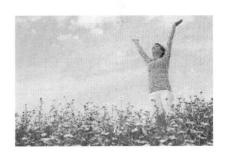

Now, take a deep breath. No, a really, *really* deep breath. Put your feet flat on the ground. Inhale through your nose as deeply as you can. Do your shoulders rise? I bet they do! Even experienced breathers fall into the habit of breathing high in their chest. Try again, put your left hand on your chest and your right hand on your abdomen. Your left hand should remain still while your right hand rises and falls. Your abdomen should fill with air and your belly should push outward. *That* is a proper deep diaphragmatic breath!

Cleansing Breath Exercise

I highly recommend practicing deep, cleansing breathing on a regular basis. The 3-3-6 Breath concentrates on ridding your lungs of every last bit of carbon dioxide while the 6-3-3 Breath concentrates on bringing as much fresh oxygenated air deep into your lungs as possible. Here is how you do it…

Phase I: The 3-3-6 Breath: Take a deep breath through your nose, deep into your lungs for a three count. Hold it for a three count. Exhale through your nose for a six count, pushing every last bit of breath out. Repeat this 10 times:

- Inhale for 3 seconds
- Hold for 3 seconds
- Exhale for 6 seconds

Now do the opposite…

Phase II: The 6-3-3 Breath: Inhale through your nose for a six count, pulling in as much air as you can, deep into your abdomen. Hold for a three count. Exhale through your mouth quickly for a 3 count, pushing the air out as fast and as hard as you can. Repeat this 10 times:

- Inhale for 6 seconds
- Hold for 3 seconds
- Exhale for 3 seconds

How does it feel to *really* fill your lungs? When you breathe deep like this, you are using your diaphragm. The diaphragm is a sheet of muscle located right beneath your lungs. When you breathe correctly, your diaphragm pulls oxygen into your lungs. Because your diaphragm is a muscle, there is the possibility for it to become inactive, therefore leading to poor health. A daily practice of deep breathing will keep your diaphragm in shape!

Breathe Quality Air

It does not do you any good to take long, deep breaths if the air you are pulling into your body is unhealthy. In addition, poor indoor air quality especially can affect your health, comfort, and ability to work. The most common causes of indoor air quality problems are not enough ventilation and lack of fresh outdoor air. The result is an excess of carbon dioxide in the air that you breathe. Are you having headaches or feeling tired? A lack of fresh, highly oxygenated outdoor air has a massive impact on you every day!

If you work or live in a building with poor indoor air quality, you may feel that the building is hot and stuffy. This is common in smaller homes with several residents and in smaller offices with many employees or many customers. You will also notice poor air quality on long drives if you keep the windows closed in your car. Have you ever rolled down the window because you were tired while driving? You may have thought you wanted the cool air to wake you up. Actually, what has happened is you (and the other people in the car) have consumed the oxygen in the vehicle and your body is sensing carbon dioxide. Instinctively, you open that window to get more oxygen.

Therefore, the answer is simple. To optimize this essential of oxygenating and energizing your body, regardless of where you are, go for a walk (or open a window) and breathe deeply!

ESSENTIAL #2: WATER

The human body is approximately 70% water by weight. You may be thinking, "Seriously?" Well yes, seriously! This water is necessary in almost every aspect of your body, its functions and your survival and comfort. Water is necessary to regulate your body's temperature, cushion your joints, lubricate your eyes, optimize your kidney function, eliminate waste, etc. If you can think of a bodily function,

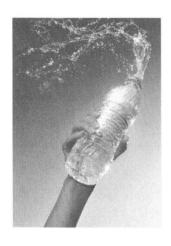

water is probably involved. Water is absolutely essential to life. You take water in mainly by eating and drinking. You breathe water out (respiration) and water evaporates through the skin (perspiration). You also lose water in your urine and waste.

If you let yourself become dehydrated for any length of time, you begin to create a toxicity crisis in your body. Heart disease, obesity, diabetes, cancer, Alzheimer's, and many other chronic forms of disease are preceded by years of not getting enough water in your system. Bacteria, viruses, and infections cannot thrive in a well-hydrated body. Therefore, drinking enough water is one of the most effective disease-prevention measures you can take.

Water and Your Kidneys

Your body has to work very hard to keep its internal body fluids at a constant concentration as well as its electrolytes in balance, but this work occurs without you even being aware of it. It needs to maintain a precise *volume* of blood, and this blood needs to be maintained at a fairly precise *concentration level*. Yet, how do you maintain the volume and concentration of blood just so? Have you ever wondered why your blood, saliva, and other body fluids are not thick like mud or thin like water? It is because your kidneys are secretly slaving away.

Let's take a look at two guys about to work out, Sam and John. Sam has not had any water and works out strenuously losing water via respiration and perspiration. Sam is becoming dehydrated, he will produce very little urine, small in volume, dark in color and the urine will have an odor. However, John has been drinking lots of water and is working out the same duration and intensity as Sam. John loses just as much water through respiration and perspiration (possibly more because he wasn't dehydrated), but John's urine will be larger in volume, clearer in color and possibly odorless. Why?

The fact that John's kidneys are releasing more urine indicates that his body is well hydrated. Kidneys regulate how much urine is produced. John's kidneys determined how much of the water consumed was necessary to keep his blood at a constant volume and concentration.

Your kidneys process your entire body's blood supply 15 times every hour. This means by the time you are 85 years old, your kidneys will have processed your entire blood supply over 10.5 million times! That is a lot of work for two little organs the size of your fist. If you are not properly hydrated, your kidneys cannot do their job properly, causing your blood volume and concentration to be compromised. The scary thought is that you could lose 90% of your kidney function before you are even aware there is anything wrong.

Let's go back to Sam and John. If they both drink a gallon of water each, Sam, who was dehydrated, would notice that he is gradually producing more urine that is getting lighter in color. This would indicate that his body is using the water to remedy the state of dehydration in his body. His blood would be able to return to a safe volume and concentration. John, who was already well hydrated, would produce close to equal the amount of urine as the gallon of water he just drank, because his body was already very close to homeostasis – which means his blood was at the correct volume and concentration for his body.

Dehydration

The best way to describe how absolutely impactful dehydration is on the overall body would be for you visualize a watermill… you know, those little buildings with a giant wheel on the side of them. The water (usually from a mill pond, stream or river) flows past the building, gets caught up in the water wheel and spins. As the volume and flow of water increases, the faster the water wheel turns. These water wheels provided energy for grinding flour, grinding pulp, or creating electricity.

Think of your body the same as a watermill. When there is a great volume of water, the water wheel turns faster and the mill produces that much more energy. When there is low or no water flow, the water wheel spins sporadically and slowly or not at all. The mill does not function at the level of efficiency it is capable of, and sometimes in the case of low or no water flow, the mill shuts down. This is precisely the impact water has on every function of your body. There is a lag time between the water wheel spinning fast and it stopping when the water flow decreases. Just as you will not feel the effects of dehydration immediately, the mill master will not be aware of the decrease in production until it is too late.

The Dehydration Test

The skin is the largest organ of the body. Did you know that medical professionals use a highly advanced scientific technique to determine if you are dehydrated? They just pinch you! Ok, so it's not so advanced, but it is extremely effective. This test is something you can do at home and it determines skin turgor. Skin turgor is a fancy name for "hey, how fast does your skin bounce back if I pull on it?"

This is how you do the skin turgor test: Lightly pinch the skin on the back of your hand between your thumb and your first finger. Pull the skin up (gently) and hold it up like a little tent. Let go. If you are well hydrated, you will have normal turgor and the skin will bounce back immediately. However, if you are dehydrated, the skin will not bounce back. In fact, it will appear to slowly collapse back into place, almost like it is slowly melting.

Because your skin is the last organ in the body to receive the nutrients you consume or the water your drink, skin turgor is considered a late sign of dehydration. Decreased skin turgor exists in *moderate to severe dehydration.*

Drink Enough Water to Keep Your Urine Clear

So how much water do you need? KEEP IT SIMPLE! The formula for the perfect amount of water for your own personal, unique need is to simply *drink enough water to keep your urine clear.* That's it.

Ok, for those who are sticklers for details wanting a formula that is more complicated... this is for you: Divide your body weight by two and drink that many ounces of water per day. For example, if you weigh 200 pounds, drink 100 ounces of water per day. If you weigh 150 pounds, drink 75 ounces of water per day.

Not complicated enough? Other factors that could be calculated into the equation are the climate you live in, the altitude, how much daily exercise, beverages with diuretic properties, and your current health status. How are you going to measure and keep track of all that? Well, every morning you could measure out your water for the day, or you could just simply *drink enough water to keep your urine clear.*

Whether you like to keep it simple or you like to measure and be precise, just know that if you are keeping water by your side, on your desk or in your car and sipping it constantly you are well on your way to giving your body what it needs. If your urine is clear, not only can you rest assured that your body has enough water to ward off a list of symptoms, but also you have enough to aid in weight loss! Keep in mind that certain medications and supplements can alter the color of the urine, which would make this method a little challenging.

Coffee, tea, milk, juice, soda, and non-fat double decaf-toffee-nut-lattes contain water but are not hydrating. Even though your body does obtain water from water-enriched foods and beverages, water should be obtained through its purest form. That is the most bioavailable form, and your body can utilize it immediately without being taxed with digestive actions.

Purpose of Thirst

The purpose of thirst is to save your life. By the time you are thirsty, your body is already in a state of moderate to severe dehydration. Thirst is not an indicator of hydration. It is an indicator of a *severe* situation in your body that needs to be fixed immediately. It is an *urgent* notification that your fluid levels are becoming *dangerously* low. In short, thirst is an indicator that your brain sends out to tell you, *"Danger! Must hydrate! Stat!"* It is not a light tap on the shoulder telling you to grab a sip of water.

Thirst is a sign that your body is going into crisis and *begging* for you to help. Never allow yourself to get thirsty.

ESSENTIAL #3: FOOD

It is ironic. We will go out of our way spending extra money to put better quality gas in our cars, yet we (as a society) are not fueling our bodies correctly.

In order to transform your health, you *must* regularly fuel yourself with the right foods. Moreover, those foods need to be as live and nutritional as possible.

Eating a steady diet of living foods not only helps you ward off illnesses and diseases, but also profoundly increases your vitality in a multitude of ways including improved heart health, brain function, bone and teeth strength, elevated energy and better weight control.

In addition, you will radiantly glow and look good!

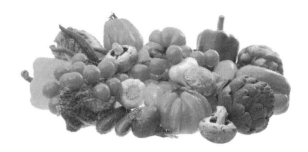

What Are Living Foods?

Living foods are plant foods such as nuts, seeds, grains, herbs, fruits, vegetables, and leafy greens that are in their natural form. They are eaten fresh (i.e. as is, cut, chopped blended or juiced – not cooked). They are packed with a wide variety of vital life force nutrients such as vitamins, minerals, amino acids, oxygen, and live enzymes that are necessary for your body to thrive.

Jay Kordich, American television personality, author, and motivational speaker known as "The Father of Juicing" and a true master of vitality, promotes that we all should be consuming nutritional, living foods. Jay just actively celebrated his 90th birthday (August 2013). He has a volume of energy, is profoundly alert and very wise.

Jay says, "Mother Nature bakes our plant foods to perfection. It is best to consume these foods with their naturally intrinsic values intact. In this way, all the life-giving vitamins, minerals and enzymes inherent in them can be absorbed."

By consuming a regular diet of foods that are fresh and living rather than cooked and processed, you become far healthier because *living foods are perfect just as they are*.

Food Toxicity

As I said earlier, we are too smart for our own good. Our power to think often overrides what our bodies are trying to tell us. As a result, we develop food intolerances without even realizing it. Processed and fast foods (which are causing a tremendous obesity crisis in our society today) are not created naturally in our environment. Your body does not know what to do with it. Your body wants to do what is right for you and will try to extract what is needed in order to do that. However, much of that is toxic and foreign substance that your body cannot use, so it remains in your body as excess gunk, much of which is stored in the form of fat.

We can all agree that processed foods are not good for you. Beyond that, there are natural foods that are considered healthy, yet may be toxic to your specific system. That is where food allergies come into play.

Food allergies can create one of the most dramatic responses of crisis in the body. For example, some people are allergic to strawberries. If a strawberry is put into the mouth of the wrong person, it can kill that person. That is the most severe form of a food allergy. You have everything from that extreme to food intolerances. Say you are lactose intolerant and you drink dairy products. You are not going to die, but your stomach will not be able to process the lactose (due to a lack of an enzyme) and you most likely will have stomach discomfort, gas and possibly diarrhea.

Those examples are some of the more common allergies and intolerances that most people know about. However, what you may not know is that there are hundreds of otherwise healthy foods that will cause reactions in your system and you may not be considering them as the cause. This is known as Immunoglobulin G (IgG) response, which causes chronic symptoms that you may be relating to other causes, when in fact, you just don't realize that the foods you are eating are the actual culprits.

95% of our population has food allergies! That means 95 people out of every 100 (or 7.6 out of 8) is allergic to one food or another. Imagine that in terms of your own family or group of friends.

When eating any foods that you are intolerant or allergic to, chronic symptoms such as chest pain, back pain, arthritis, rashes, or even lung issues such as asthma can result. We tend to think of asthma as something caused by the air that you breath, but it can literally be caused by foods that you are eating.

People who are having issues with weight loss, weight gain, or think they are doing all of the right things and eating all of the right foods are in actuality eating foods that are not compatible with their specific systems. Many of the chronic symptoms that people are experiencing such as anxiety, irritability, depression, and nervousness may all be secondary reactions to food intolerances or food allergies. How about headaches, insomnia, memory loss, poor concentration, or brain fog? For a more intensive list of symptoms caused by foods, take a look at the Physicians Test Indicator Guide located in Appendix A on page 137.

Once I became clear about what I wanted for my health and vitality, I prioritized what I wanted most, to get down to my ideal body weight and to get rid of the chronic pain I was experiencing. When I wrote down all of my goals, getting rid of pain in my body was on top of the list, even above financial gain. That sent a clear message to me how debilitating that pain had become in my life. I had to take a look at what it was that I was doing to my body to cause this. Of course, being a doctor, I did many assessments. The results were improper structural alignment, food intolerances (of over 20 foods) and hormonal imbalances.

Before Starting a New Program, Consult Your Doctor. I am sure you have heard this before. Well, it is wise. Before you start taking supplements, pain killers, changing your diet, or going to the gym, it is smart to find out what is going on with you that needs to be corrected. All of these things are helpful, but there may be an easier fix.

I wanted to find the simple fixes by first getting a blood test to find out where I was (clarity) and see if anything was biochemically out of balance. Much to my surprise, I found that my testosterone was low! With low testosterone, you can have the exact symptoms that I was having (chronic pain, sore muscles, decreased flexibility, increased joint pain, rapid aging, thinning of the skin, decreased stamina, and an overall burnt-out feeling). I had every single one of those symptoms.

Hormone Imbalance

I am going to take a moment to talk about hormones because this goes hand-in-hand with your food intake and how this can affect your vitality. All of your hormones (estrogen, progesterone, testosterone), as well as cholesterol (an important hormonal precursor which aides in hormonal function) and your thyroid gland (which produces hormones) need to be in balance. I have patients who complain about symptoms all the time, and they believe that it is normal to tolerate them because they have had them for years. However, they can have something as simple as adrenal fatigue or low cortisone levels, which are easy to fix. In most cases, their medications were suppressing the symptoms, not addressing the *source* of the problem in the first place! Symptoms are the way our bodies yell at us for help. When we mask our symptoms with medications, we are just turning down the volume. You wouldn't do that if a child was screaming for help, would you?

The following is a list of symptoms that can be caused by your hormones being out of balance (Take note if any of these apply to you):

- Aches and pains
- Acne
- Allergies
- Anxiety
- Bone loss
- Breast tenderness
- Cold body temperature
- Decreased libido
- Decreased muscle size
- Decreased stamina
- Depression
- Difficulty sleeping
- Dizzy spells
- Dry or brittle hair
- Fatigue
- Fibroids
- Fibromyalgia
- Foggy thinking
- Hair loss
- Headaches
- Heart palpitations
- High cholesterol
- Hot flashes
- Incontinence
- Increased facial and body hair
- Increased urinary urge
- Infertility problems
- Irregular bleeding (menstrual)
- Irregular heart beat
- Irritability
- Mental fatigue
- Mood swings
- Morning fatigue
- Nervousness
- Night sweats
- Prostate problems,
- Rapid aging
- Rapid or slow pulse rate
- Ringing in the ears
- Stress
- Sugar cravings
- Tearfulness
- Thinning of the skin
- Vaginal dryness
- Water retention
- Weight gain (especially in the hips, waist or chest)

There are simple ways to get your hormones back in balance through change in diet, life-style, or hormonal replacement if necessary. Regardless of the direction you choose to correct your symptoms, you cannot do that successfully unless you first identify the actual cause. The way for you to do that is to be tested.

It is always wise to get a baseline to know where you are. Blood Chemistry Test, Lipid Panel, Comprehensive Hormone Panel and Food Allergy Panel (both immediate & delayed reactivity) – these are tests I recommend that you get done for yourself (by a licensed professional) as soon as possible. You are welcome to contact us at *MasteringVitalityNow.com* and have us guide you through the process.

Identifying food toxicity, food intolerances, food allergies, and hormonal imbalances along with issues in structural alignment, can make the difference between why you might have depression, chronic pain, chronic conditions, problems losing weight or are on certain medications. This is very easy to identify, and it is reversible.

The 70/30 Rule

Now let's go back to what you eat. Overall, a diet that is primarily plant-based is the key to preventing many diseases such as heart disease, diabetes, and cancer. Of course, it is also key to controlling weight, feeling youthful and charging your energy. Therefore, when you fill up your plate, there should be at least 70% fresh fruits and vegetables, of which need to be as raw and organic as possible. Think dark green, dark orange and red first, then fill in the rest of the 70% with leafy greens, natural herbs and spices.

The remaining 30% of your plate is everything else. Yes, everything else. This 30% includes proteins such as chicken, tofu, nuts, seeds, or seafood. It also includes any dairy such as butter, milk, cream, or cheese. Yes, this same 30% includes any "cheat" treats such as candies, chocolate, or caffeine. There are many theories about what the 30% should or should not contain. Whether you are a meat eater or Vegan, do not get caught up on the 30% so much that you lose focus on the 70%. Remember, whether you are correct or incorrect on the 30%, the consequences become less important as long as 70% of your intake is live fruits and vegetables.

Whether you are correct or incorrect on the 30%, the consequences become less important as long as 70% of your intake is live fruits and vegetables. Once you have mastered the 70%, then you can further improve upon the 30%. Once you have mastered the 70%, then you can further improve upon the 30%.

Local Foods

Your body is designed to benefit from food that is closer to the source in which it was grown because it has less travel time, is allowed to naturally ripen, and is exposed to fewer chemicals. This means it is less likely that the nutritional values have dropped. In addition, the more your food is handled, the more chances there are for contamination.

Local plant and animal foods are generated from similar soil, water, and air, and share the same climatic conditions. Thus, they are uniquely adapted to support the life of their area's inhabitants. For this reason, it is recommend that 90% of your diet comes from your own region (loosely defining "region" as within a 300 to 500 mile radius encompassing all areas with similar environmental patterns).

Besides that, local foods taste better! Most are picked within 24 hours of you purchasing them. This means that instead of being harvested early in order to be shipped and distributed to your local retail store, the crops can be picked at their peak of ripeness.

There are many other benefits of buying local foods, such as to help keep the money within your community and conserve energy by decreasing the need for transportation. The bottom line is, the more you can close the gap between you and where your food originates, the more you are doing yourself a great favor.

Juicing

Most every food you can think of has come under some criticism, except fruits and vegetables. These foods are packed with vitamins and minerals, hydrate and nourish every cell in your body, prevent diseases, flush your system of waste, reduce inflammation, help you lose weight, and much more. By juicing, you get a quick, efficient way to maximize getting high-value nutrients into your body and instantly reverse the ill effects of poor diet. NOTE: It is best when making fresh juices to drink them within the hour so that you don't lose these precious enzymes vital to building energy and superior digestion.

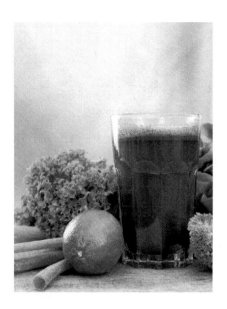

In his book, *Jay Kordich's Live Food, Live Bodies*, Jay tells us that the real advantage of fresh, live juice is that you have a powerhouse rich in vitamins, minerals, live enzymes, and phytochemicals; all of which have an extraordinarily healthful and beneficial effect on your body. Another man, who is crucial in the history and development of juicing, is Dr. Max Gerson. Dr. Gerson is profiled in a wildly successful documentary, *The Beautiful Truth*. Dr. Gerson is the physician who treated Jay Kordich for bladder cancer back in 1947. Jay was only 25 years old and a strong football player for USC when he became injured and was diagnosed. He had the option of having a year to live or receiving surgery and going through cobalt treatments. Jay heard of Dr. Gerson who was known for treating cancer with what was referred to in Europe as "Juice Therapy". After juicing for what Jay refers to as a "grueling" program for 3 months and continuing on a live foods program for another 2 years, Jay's cancer was gone.

You are very fortunate today because juicing has become popular. Recipes, blogs, and articles about juicing are easily found on the Internet. In most cities, you can find several juice bars, and in most health food stores you can purchase fresh juice or even have some made especially for you.

It is best to pick out your fruits and vegetables yourself and buy as local and organic as possible. Whichever you do, make it easy and convenient. Mastering Vitality is about making simple, lifelong changes that are enjoyable.

Supplements

You may be wondering, "Are supplements really necessary?" I am here to tell you that supplements are definitely helpful, especially with today's diet. In America, we are vitamin and mineral depleted and have hormonal deficiencies, so supplements are definitely helpful. However, they are not absolutely necessary. You do not need to be caught up in that obstacle of thinking.

The closer that you can be to the way that nature intended, the better. Whole foods are God's foods. And as we discussed above, eating live foods that will give you energy, vitamins and minerals – is what's ideal. If you think that you are vitamin deficient, then your primary care physician or certified nutrition specialist should be able to help you.

Best Eating Habits

As much as possible, you want to be on a living foods, raw, plant-based diet. I cannot stress that enough. Typically, what you hear is correct: keep it low salt, low fat, and low cholesterol. What you eat is important, and *how* you eat is just as important. Below is a list of eating tips that I have found to be most useful.

Listen to your body. Have you ever felt bloated after eating? Sluggish? Tired? Or do you just have that super full feeling? These are signs that you either ate the wrong thing, or you ate too much. Make sure that you stay tuned-in, listen to your body and adjust accordingly. Your body is pretty smart.

Make a list first! Go to the grocery store with a purpose and stay focused. Stock up on food that is going to help you meet your goals. If you predetermine what you are going to get before you leave, not only will you be there a shorter amount of time, but you will also make better choices.

Never, *ever* go grocery shopping while you are hungry. If you get hungry and go grocery shopping, you will end up with an abundance of items in your cart that you have never purchased before just because they look good! Also, stay on the perimeter; this is where all of the healthy stuff located. You want to stay away from the items in the middle isles… the processed foods. Chips, crackers, sodas, candy, and the like are all in the middle section. Stay out – that is a danger zone!

Set yourself up to win. The last thing that you want is a bunch of unhealthy foods staring at you. Clear out your refrigerator and cupboards from all temptations. Those "temptations" eventually end up in the sewer anyway – so don't run it through your body first! Pre-cut live foods (such as fruits and vegetables) and keep salads and other healthy treats on hand for you to enjoy. If you have snacks for kids or other members in your household, put them in a different section of the kitchen where you won't see them. You don't have to transform your entire house/kitchen, just your section. Make sure you are setting yourself up to win.

Eat frequent meals. A lot of times people starve themselves all day, thinking that they are doing the right thing, but then when they do eat, they eat tons of food. Yet, the design of your body is to be fueled a little bit at a time throughout the day. Make sure you are eating small, frequent meals. This will speed up your metabolism as well and help you to lose weight.

Chew your food! Digesting your food begins in your mouth. Chewing breaks down your food so that it can be easily digested thus making it easier for your intestines to absorb the necessary nutrients. The longer you chew, the slower you will eat, which also helps with weight loss. In addition, as you shift your diet to 70 percent live foods, chewing helps minimize the gas you may experience while making the transition. Take small bites and chew until your food has lost all of its texture. If you find being consistent with this difficult, don't worry, you just haven't developed the habit yet. Keep practicing. Take your time, relax and enjoy your food.

Keep a photo journal. If you really want to analyze whether you are getting all the nutrients you need, ask yourself if you have awareness of what you are eating, 27-7. Do you know everything that passes your lips in any given day? Keeping a photo journal is helpful – taking a photo of everything you eat in a day will give you an awareness of what is going into your body and may help you answer some questions about vitamin deficiencies. You will be surprised at some of the foods that you eat!

Eat for tomorrow. Think about the consequences of *everything* that you put into your mouth. What you eat today will show up on your body tomorrow, next week or even months from now. If you eat something healthy now, it will show up healthy later. If you eat something junky just to satisfy your taste buds, the consequence is it will show up junky on your body later. Remember, you are what you eat! So think about every bite or sip you take and make it count. You are feeding for *your future*!

Stay away from prepared foods. Most all prepared foods (processed and packaged) have "bad" calories that can add to your caloric intake. They have been stripped of the many important nutrients that you need. In addition, most are filled with sugars, salts, and chemicals that are harmful to your body. The closer you can get to the natural source of your food the better.

Get rid of the condiments and spices, especially sugar and salt. You do not need them. Many foods already have natural sugars and salts in them and are rich in their own flavors. Over time, our taste buds get down-regulated, so it takes more salt to make something taste salty and more sugar to make something taste sweet. As you cut these things out of your diet, your taste buds will up-regulate and fewer of these things will be needed to get the same result.

Always be relaxed when you eat. Stress creates cortisol, the "fight or flight" hormone that tells your body to hold on to or store calories/glucose just in case you need it in a stressful situation. If you are relaxed while you eat, that is going to aid in your weight-loss. When you are stressed or when you are trying to multi-task (eating while checking emails, on the run, etc.), your body will hold on to the weight because it believes it will need the calories. Eating should be a relaxed, enjoyable process.

ESSENTIAL #4: MOVEMENT

Before you read this chapter, stand up and shake your body out. Stretch to the left, stretch to the right and then jump up and down a few times. I'm serious – get up right now and do it! You will thank me for it. There, now don't you feel better? Perhaps a little more energized? (You're welcome!)

You body is meant to move. As human beings, we evolved to stand upright and move, and historically our environment demanded us to be physically active. Yet today, as more and more modern conveniences are developed along with the technological advances of the Internet, you can literally get anything you need without so much as leaving your computer chair. Studies show that, on average, nearly half of our waking time is spent being sedentary. The problem with that is when you sit for extended periods of time, your body starts to shut down at the metabolic level, which leads to numerous serious health issues including weight gain and depression.

The experience of movement is highly beneficial in so many ways: physically, preventively, emotionally, mentally, psychologically, and spiritually. Movement encourages your lymphatic flow thus improving your immune system, which in turn helps you fight off illnesses and diseases. It increases circulation to 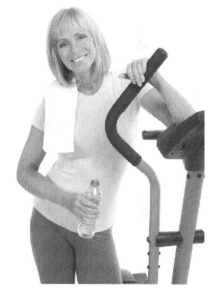 deliver nutrients, oxygen, and water throughout your body. It strengthens your heart and keeps your body flexible and strong. Movement provides more oxygen to your brain and increases brain function so that you can think more clearly. It releases endorphins that make you feel happier. It helps "burn off" anger and frustration. It energizes you. It increases your desire for sex, and makes you more attractive to other people. Movement is free, readily available, within your control and the single most impactful way to influence your health and fitness.

Be proactive in finding ways to keep your body moving. Find something fun to do for 30 minutes a day to get your heart rate up. I'm sure you can think of something. The key is having fun while you are doing it!

Aerobic vs. Anaerobic Activity

It is important to understand the difference between aerobic and anaerobic activity. Basically, aerobic activity is anything that gets your heart rate and respiration up. However, anaerobic is high-intensity activity, where your body's demand for oxygen exceeds the oxygen supply available. Anaerobic activity means without oxygen. You do not want to be anaerobic for too long or it could end up being your last activity… possibly for your life. So, make it your goal to stay aerobic.

Always pay attention to what your body is feeling. You should not feel any pain while exercising. If you do feel any pain, it is time to stop. If you are having chest pain, severe back pain, or something that you are unsure of, contact your physician.

Heart Rate

Your heart rate is defined by how many times your heart beats in one minute. In order to know that you are moving at an aerobic pace that is right for you, it is important to know your heart rate. The easiest way is to check this is to count the number of beats per second in the carotid artery (neck), or your radial (wrist) pulse. A quicker way is to count the number of beats in 10 seconds and multiply that number by six, or count the number of beats in 30 seconds and multiply that number by two. Either way, that will give you your heart rate (also known as your pulse).

Next, you need to know what your Maximum Aerobic Heart Rate

should be while you are exercising. This number depends on your age. To determine this, simply subtract your age from the number 220. That will be your Maximum Aerobic Heart Rate. For example, the average 60 year old would take 220 minus 60 and get 160. While exercising, their heart rate should not go above 160 beats per minute.

220 (minus your age) = Your **Maximum Aerobic Heart Rate** per minute

Another good formula to know is 180 minus your age. This will give you your Ideal Aerobic Heart Rate while exercising to get the maximum aerobic benefit. So to use the previous example, the average 60 year old should have a Maximum Aerobic Heart Rate of 160, and an average Ideal Aerobic Heart Rate of 120.

180 (minus your age) = Your **Ideal Aerobic Heart Rate** per minute

If you are someone who works out regularly, you can add about 10 beats to that, however that number is still going to fall into that range because the more in shape you are, the lower your heart rate becomes.

Your resting heart rate should be between 60 and 80 beats per minute. If you live a sedentary lifestyle (meaning that you are pretty much a couch potato) that number may be a little elevated. If you are older, that number might be a little elevated as well. It should always be less than 100 beats per minute. A top athlete will have a resting heart rate of around 60 beats per minute. What this means is that the athlete's heart is strong enough to pump blood sufficiently throughout the entire body at only 60 beats per minute

You should now be able to tell what your resting heart rate, maximum heart rate and what your ideal aerobic heart rate should be.

Set Yourself up to Win!

Start slow. A big reason that people stop or lose focus is because they bite off more than they can chew, they become discouraged, and then they quit. That is not something you want to set yourself up for.

Start slow and simple. Make sure you do not have to jump over a bunch of obstacles in order to get going. You do not need to join a gym, pay a personal trainer, or buy fancy equipment. Those are obstacles that could potentially set you up for failure. Find something that is easy to do, and most importantly make it fun! If it's fun, it's sustainable!

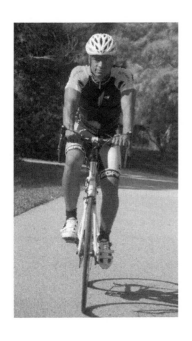

Make it fun. My motto is: "If it's not fun, don't do it!" Instead of thinking about exercising, think about doing *fun aerobic movement*. If you like dancing, then dance! If you like walking, then walk! If you like running, then run! If you don't like going to the gym and running on the treadmill, then consider doing something else like riding your bike, playing with your dog or chasing children or grand children. (They would love that!) Maybe pick a sport you like. Even gardening works. The point is for you to get moving and do something every day that is both enjoyable and beneficial to your health.

Assess your current fitness level. And I mean your *current* fitness level, not where you were ten years ago. You do not want to hurt yourself and you certainly do not want to set yourself up for failure. Get out and do something you know that you can do. Walk a mile, or walk up and down some flights of stairs. Map out a route and time yourself. How long can you walk? How long did it take? How many flights of stairs can you do without getting extremely short of breath? Write it down, and then your *only goal* is to do a little better each time. *Remember, small steps taken consistently over a long period of time produce extraordinary results!*

Get clear on your outcome. What do you want to accomplish? Write your fitness goals on a piece of paper and keep them in front of you so that you can stay focused. It needs to be something you can measure as well as something you can attain.

You know you want to get fit, but getting fit is not a goal; it is a mere want or a desire. Instead, focus on a *specific* activity in which you want to participate. If running is something you enjoy, find the next 5k run in your community. Set a deadline. Make a commitment to participate.

Continue working your movement plan with *consistency*. Measure your progress. Mark your milestones and celebrate them! Before you know it, your desire to get fit will be realized.

Make movement a part of your lifestyle. The best way to increase your daily movement is to make it a part of your lifestyle. Make it your identity. Movement is a sign of youth and the more you move, the more youthful you become. Have you ever noticed how children rarely stay still?

There is an unlimited amount of movement you can add to your daily activity without taking up any more of your time. For example, whenever you get out of bed, try bouncing up and down and hopping to the bathroom. Sway your hips back and forth, as you brush your teeth. Do squats while waiting for your coffee or tea. Stand up taller, breathe deeper and lengthen your stride as you walk to your car, or anywhere for that matter. Do tummy-tucks and buttock squeezes and rock out to your favorite tunes while sitting at the stop lights. Park further away and take the stairs rather than elevators. Take every opportunity to stretch and shake yourself out like you did at the start of this chapter. (You did do that, right?) Use some form of movement as a way of marking the completion of something, such as the end of every hour or the end of reading each chapter in this book!

By adding more movement to everything you do, you will find that you will have more energy to do more. It really is that simple. If you want more energy, create it! Get moving!

ESSENTIAL #5: REST

Being well rested and getting enough sleep is critical to the health and safety of every aspect of your life. It is when you sleep that your body has a chance to recharge, rejuvenate, and heal itself. Sleep deficiency can harm you in an instant by causing you to have an accident, or it can harm you over time by raising your risk for chronic health 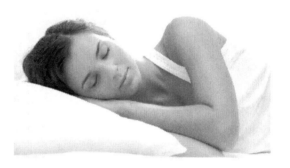 problems. Heart disease, diabetes, and obesity have all been linked with chronic sleep loss.

Studies show that there is an increased mortality risk for people getting less than six or seven hours of sleep per night. Actually, one study found that reduced sleep time is a greater mortality risk than smoking, high blood pressure, and heart disease! To say the least, getting a good night's sleep is just as important for your overall health as everything else we have talked about. If you are not getting full night, restful sleep, then try implementing the following tips into your routine.

Best Sleeping Habits

Get Up and Go To Bed at the Same Time Daily. Your body has a regular rhythm and it is best to allow your body to function how it expects to, including time for rest. It is best to set your internal clock by getting up and going to bed at the same time every day, even on weekends. If you feel like treating yourself by sleeping in, only sleep for an additional 30 minutes so that your internal clock maintains its rhythm.

Develop Sleep Rituals. Your mind and body responds to cues. When you are winding down for the day, have a ritual to trigger your mind and body to start relaxing. Your bedroom should be your sanctuary. The goal is to provide a peaceful environment where you can rest and properly program your unconscious mind (which is much more powerful than you realize). The things that you read, hear, watch, or focus on right before falling asleep are what your unconscious mind will process for the next eight hours. Be sure to feed your unconscious mind properly and help it to work for you rather than against you.

Use Sunlight to Set Your Biological Clock. I love going camping, sleeping out doors, and waking up at sunrise feeling completely rested, refreshed and full of vitality. This happens because your body is in rhythm with the earth and sunlight. At night there is no artificial environment (TV, lights, music) telling your body to stay awake, so your body is able to naturally wind down and relax. In the morning, you are surrounded by thousands of life forms celebrating the day; the sun is rising, and your body receives a gentle message to "Get up." Try to create a sleeping and waking ritual that allows your body to respond to nature and natural cues such as sunlight.

If You Can't Fall Asleep, Get Up and Do Something Boring. Do not lie in bed tossing and turning while trying to force yourself to sleep. If you've been awake for an hour, then get up and do something really boring like reading a warranty manual or scrubbing the floor with a toothbrush. Your brain will not want to do this, so chances are it will shut itself down. This does not mean you should go watch an action film. The idea is to quiet the mind. Another trick known to work is to imagine the absolute worst, most horrific, gruesome things possible. Again, your brain will refuse to go there and would rather fall asleep than think about it.

Get Plenty of Exercise Daily. Be sure to spend time during the day to exhaust your physical body. One of the primary reasons you cannot get to sleep at night is because you have not burned off the energy you have consumed throughout the day. Those calories (units of energy) are waiting to be used. If you are not physically tired, your body will utilize those calories by keeping your mind stimulated. So, be sure to exercise enough during the day to get a good night's sleep.

Refrain from Taking Naps. If you want to absolutely guarantee you won't be able to sleep at night, then wake up really late in the morning or take naps during the day. This only confuses your internal clock. One should sleep in minimum blocks of 3 hours. A nap for 3 hours in the middle of the day will regenerate your body so much that there will be no need for sleep at bedtime. Additionally, a nap shorter than 3 hours will leave your body more tired than before you napped. If you get sleepy during the day, it is best to do something physical. Breathe deep, move your body, and then go to bed at your regular bedtime. If you must nap, make it 20 minutes or less and between the hours of 1:00 to 4:00 PM so that you minimize the disruption to your sleep at night.

Refrain from "Exercise" Just Before Bedtime. The body receives so many benefits from a consistent, invigorating physical routine. However, it is best to be active in the morning to stimulate the body, its metabolism and clear your head for the day, or in the afternoon for the same reasons and to relieve stress. Avoid too much physical activity just before bedtime as it will get you stimulated and make it more difficult to fall asleep.

Avoid Caffeine, Nicotine, and Alcohol 4-6 Hours Before Bedtime.
If you go to bed at 11PM, make a rule that you don't drink any type of caffeine after 5 or 6PM. Coffee, tea, soda, cocoa, and some drugs (prescription and non-prescription) contain caffeine. Alcohol may appear to help you fall asleep, but you will experience fragmented sleep. In general, I would say avoid all nicotine and alcohol, period. However, if you are not yet ready to quit cold turkey at this time, then at least stay away from these substances at least 4-6 hours before your bedtime. A warm cup of herbal tea is a nice alternative to caffeinated beverages.

Have a Light Snack. If you are hungry when you go to bed, it will be difficult to sleep. On the other hand, if you just ate a huge meal, it will also be difficult to sleep. Dairy products and turkey contain tryptophan, which acts as a natural sleep inducer. (Remember all of those lazy Thanksgiving afternoons?) This is why a warm glass of milk at bedtime has traditionally done the trick. This bedtime ritual could also be duplicated with a non-dairy product such as rice milk, coconut milk, almond milk, or soymilk. It isn't just the tryptophan that assisted sleep; it is the ritual of enjoying a warm beverage before bedtime.

Take a Hot Bath. Getting in a hot bath will raise your body temperature, but it is the drop in temperature after you get out that makes you sleepy. Take a nice hot bath 90 minutes before bedtime. Make it a ritual; add a candle or essential oil and some calming music.

Make Your Bedroom Comfortable. Create a space that is comfortable and free of clutter so that you can let your mind go. If your bedroom is too hot or too cold, it will be difficult to sleep. Keeping your bedroom a bit on the cool side with warm blankets is recommended. If you are sensitive to light and have street lamps near you, get a black-out shade. Conversely, if you are a heavier sleeper and alarms do not seem to work, open your shades at night and allow the sun to assist you in starting your day.

Make sure you have a comfortable bed and a proper pillow. You spend nearly a third of your life asleep, and most of that time, you spend in bed. Your body benefits more from a good bed and pillow than a nice car, so invest in a great mattress and pillow. It is worth it for a good night's sleep and all of the benefits mentioned above.

Rest well and enjoy sweet dreams!

ESSENTIAL #6: SEX

Sex. Need I say more? My guess is the very thought of it has changed your state. Sex is as natural as eating and sleeping or singing

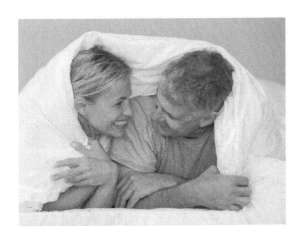

in the shower. It blurs the lines between your physical body, mental awareness, emotional fortitude, and spiritual depth. Without sex, life as we know it would not exist.

Aside from the obvious benefits from increasing your heart rate (as we talked about in Essential #4: Movement), having a healthy sex life can provide some incredible boosts to your overall well-being and quality of life. Because sex is linked to love and power as well as morality, it can also have a profound effect on how you view it emotionally. If this is a difficult subject for you, I suggest you explore it further with the help of a professional. As I said, it is as natural as eating and sleeping, and the benefits to your health are plentiful.

Benefits of Sex

Lower Blood Pressure. Research suggests that there is a link between sex and lower blood pressure, which in turn lowers your chance of developing heart disease, stroke, and other serious conditions.

Relieves Stress. Having sexual intercourse triggers the release of hormones, such as cortisol and epinephrine, which help you to feel calm and at ease as well as boost your sense of pleasure and self-esteem. Research also shows that people who have sex regularly tend to be more confident in public.

Elevates Mood and Bonding. Scientists from Rutgers University found that up to 30 different parts of the woman's brain is activated during orgasm, including those responsible for emotion, touch, joy and satisfaction.

Improves Long-Term Memory. Dopamine, also known as the "feel-good" hormone, is released during sexual activity and improves your long-term memory.

Improves Sleep. Again, hormones are released during sex. Prolactin helps you fall asleep, and oxytocin, known as the "love hormone" not only creates a sense of bonding, but also helps to promote sleep. This means you will most likely fall asleep with a smile on your face.

Minimizes Pain. The pain-reducing hormones released during sex have been found to reduce back and leg pain as well as pain from arthritis, menstruation, and headaches (including migraines). So if your partner says, "Not tonight, I have a headache," now you know how you can help!

Boosts Immune System. If you have sex more than one or two times a week, studies show that you will have significantly higher levels of immunoglobulin A (IgA), which is your body's first line of defense against invading organisms. This is an excellent way for you to reduce your chances of catching the common cold. Viva la IgA!

Heart Health. If you are a man who is having sex at least twice a week, according to some studies, you are 45% less likely to develop heart disease than your brother who is only doing it once a month or less.

Boosts Your Libido. The more you have sex, the more likely you will want to keep doing it. The hormones released in your body not only elevate how you feel physically and mentally, but also they make the very act of sex itself more pleasurable by increasing vaginal lubrication, blood flow and elasticity.

Reduces Risk of Prostate Cancer. Men who ejaculate a minimum of 21 times per month have a lower risk of developing prostate cancer. In other words, if you don't use it, you lose it – so use it!

Bladder Control. For women, regular orgasms help to strengthen the pelvic floor, which in turn, means lowering your chances of becoming incontinent, especially during sex.

Increased Intimacy and Improved Relationships. Increased levels of oxytocin help you to feel more bonded to your partner. You will experience a closer connection, not only emotionally, but also physically-bonded and mentally-connected.

Physically Toned. On average, sex burns between 125 – 300 calories per hour. The cardio benefits of having sex are great for toning your muscles and increasing your metabolism, which in turn helps you to keep your body energetic and lean.

Youthful Appearance. Having sex promotes the release of hormones, including testosterone and estrogen, which help to keep the body looking young. Estrogen promotes soft skin and shiny hair. One study showed that those who were enjoying ample sex with a steady partner on a regular basis were perceived to be seven to twelve years younger than their actual age!

So the moral of this story is, get your sexy on!

ESSENTIAL #7: SPIRIT

Over 2,400 years ago, the great philosopher Plato Aristocles wrote, "No attempt should be made to cure the body without curing the soul." When I speak of spirit, I speak of life energy and its relation to your soul.

Of all the Seven Essentials, spirit is the most abstract because it differs from person to person in beliefs. In this section, I will address both the tangible and intangible aspects of this essential part of your life.

Even though the concept of spirituality is intangible, science is able to prove that it can have a very tangible and measurable benefit to your health. Researchers have found that people who meditate, pray or practice some sort of religious or spiritual connection tend to live happier and healthier lives.

Please know that I am not here to tell you what you should believe. That is not my purpose. Your reality is for you to determine. My purpose is to give you all of the tools you need to master vitality so that you can live in optimum health in *every* aspect of your life, including your soul. So let's take a look at the connection between the powers of spirituality and its impact on the wholeness of human wellness.

Connection

We are all spiritual beings. Our bodies grow, function, maintain, and repair themselves without us even having to think about it. Babies are born, thunderstorms strike and flowers bloom. Who's running the show? Whether you are religious, spiritual, or neither, I think we can all agree (even Albert Einstein) that there are miracles in life that just cannot be explained. Our existence is one of them. And even though we apparently cannot bring ourselves into existence, we can certainly create a life of vitality that is deeply fulfilling and highly meaningful by simply understanding the connection we have with life energy, also known as spirit.

Everything in our bodies works together like a sophisticated symphony, from complex systems and organs to tiny cells and particles. The conductor is our brain, firing electrifying messages to keep our bodies alive and well. When everything in your body is working as intended, you are physically healthy. When your mind is in harmony with your outside world, you are mentally healthy. When you have a connection between your body, mind and soul as well as the life source that created our universe, then you my friend, are spiritually healthy.

The question of life source is never more obvious than in the moment this spirit leaves the body. As a hospitalist, I see people at some of the worst moments in their lives such as when they have lost a limb, been diagnosed with a life-threatening disease or just lost someone they truly loved. It is times like these that people connect even deeper with the spirit in which they believe.

We are all a part of the same universe. Just as your body is interconnected within you, you are interconnected with your outside world and those around you. We travel this journey called "life" together – each of us in our own way, our own time and with our own perspectives. It is natural for us to desire connection with each other as well as a higher power. Some of the best ways I have found to do that is with regular practice of faith and meditation, prayer or even yoga.

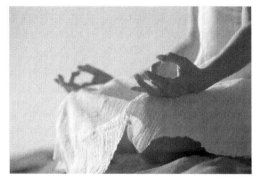

There is a blurred line between the definition of meditation and prayer, depending on what your ultimate beliefs are about connection with spirit. Crossover between the two exists, and people have different approaches to both. For the purposes of this book, I will classify meditation as more of a deliberate *silence* and prayer as more of a deliberate *communication*.

Meditation

I heard it said that meditation is the sound of one hand clapping. The intention is to quiet your mind and experience your core nature, which is described as peace, happiness, joy and bliss. A common misconception is that you need to sit in an uncomfortable position on the floor and try to get all thoughts out of your head. This is why most people fail after trying for a short period of time, or won't try it at all. I love the scene in the 2010 film *Eat, Pray, Love* where Elizabeth Gilbert (played by Julia Roberts) is staring at the clock and every sound is getting exponentially louder. It is a hilarious example of the pressure we put on ourselves while trying to do everything perfect. The art of meditation is not about trying to get it perfect.

Meditation is a practice that has been around for thousands of years and there are many different forms. Knowing which one is right for you can be difficult. I encourage you to meditate (if you are not already doing so). There are so many benefits that range from calming and healing physical, emotional, and mental stress to experiencing higher levels of consciousness and achieving self-realization through connecting with a universal wisdom. All of these will help you to increase healthiness in mind, body, and soul.

No matter how you meditate, once you start you will experience the benefits. Don't worry about the silence, the music, the incense or whether you are meditating while sitting up, lying down, walking or running. Find a way that works for you and enjoy the experience.

Prayer

In a Pennsylvanian laboratory, a Presbyterian minister sat in a state of deep, silent prayer. She was well experienced at the art of praying since she had been religiously doing it daily for over 34 years. This time, as she reached the height of connection with God, neurologist Andrew Newberg injected a harmless radioactive dye into her arm. As she continued to pray, the dye migrated to the parts of her brain where the blood flow was the strongest.

"The more active a particular part of the brain is," Dr. Newberg tells us, "the more blood flow it gets. The less active it is, the less blood flow it gets."

The brain scan showed increased activity in the frontal lobes and language area of the minister's brain. This is what happens. More blood flow in any area of your body makes it healthier. When you meditate or pray, you literally make your brain healthier. The frontal lobe, which is very active when you are engaged in a conversation, also allows you to listen and speak. This means you can increase your communicative skills with regular meditation or prayer.

A video of this study can be seen courtesy of the Science Channel online. What I found particularly interesting was that the brains of meditators, who were believers in a spiritual power, had more brain activity than in the brains of meditating atheists. Dr. Newberg theorizes that this is because to an atheist, God is unimaginable. To a believer, experiences of God are more than just thoughts and are just as real as the physical world that we all sense, therefore the experience is neurologically real.

Our brain is where reality becomes crystalized for us. If you focus on a belief, your brain perceives it as real and then sends signals throughout your body to act on those thoughts. The deeper you go into meditative prayer, *and* the more spiritually connected you are, the more intensely you can neurologically increase the health of your brain as well as your reality. This is an important point because as you seek to transform your body and health, you can literally reprogram your brain through the activity of spiritually-charged meditative prayer.

Over 85% of people confronting a major illness pray.
Increasingly, evidence is showing that prayer works. Many studies are being performed to uncover the mystery of how this is possible. Although it is yet to be fully explained scientifically, it is fair to say that most people pray because we feel a connection to spirit and we believe that praying will work. The core of what we have working for us when we pray is faith.

Trying to explain the spiritual world in a scientific manner is man's desire to make the unknown, known. The result of prayer, or connecting with spirit, is certainly tangible when you see what it does for your body. However, what spirit actually *is* is intangible. True faith in spirit is giving up that expectation to be able to put God in a box. It is the act of believing in something that you cannot explain or do not fully understand, yet you trust that it is present and at work. It is like having the faith that your blood cells are flowing to all parts of your body even though you may not understand how they are working. We do not understand why the earth is rotating, but we have faith that it is.

Deepak Chopra talks about how once people are given a diagnosis and accept that reality as being true, there are certain things that happen in your body that propagate the actual belief. Prayer and faith together allows you to create a different belief that propels you in the direction of that belief. If you believe you are a person who gets sick regularly, or if you believe that you have a weak immune system, that will set off a chain of events in your body making those beliefs true.

The opposite of this is focusing on what you want rather than what you are afraid of. There is something about that belief and that focus when it pertains to your health. If you have been overweight all of your life and you have beliefs that you always will be, then focus on visualizing yourself in the body of your ideal weight and you will make that reality come true. If you have an illness, put yourself in a state where you actually visualize and believe that the illness is going away. The more you faithfully meditate and pray, the more you will increase the healing process and bring your mind, body and soul into harmonious health.

Yoga

To the mainstream, yoga may be considered mere exercise. However, in my observation, yoga cultivates life balance, flexibility and strength as well as a connection to life energy. Life energy that is strong makes you feel totally vibrant and alive while weak life energy makes you feel dull and fatigued. The essence of yoga is a union between your mind, body and soul and can serve as a spiritual connection as well, which as you read about in mediation and prayer above, serves to increase your overall health.

The practice of yoga includes simple meditation, stretching, holding specific bodily postures and breath control. There is certainly no downside to adding this type of movement to your routine. It is thought to open up the energy centers in your body, known as chakras, so that life energy (or spirit) can freely flow. If you have a clinical mind, you could find many correlations between the chakras and the physical body's systems, organs and functions.

I encourage you to practice some form of yoga and take actions to keep your chakras clear. This can be accomplished by breathing deeply into every cell of your body, exhaling fully, speaking your truth, living an authentic life, connecting to the ones you love and the nature around you, and being open to the power of the ultimate, universal connection that we all share.

Belief

We are All Spiritual Beings. The question of soul, spirit or life energy has been around for centuries and always comes back to what you believe. Everyone's belief system is personal. I respect whatever your personal connection is and fully support your journey to wholeness. I believe that we are all connected and are one in the same universe. I am so very grateful for you and celebrate that you are answering this calling to master your vitality. Just as blood magically flowed to the minister's brain, and the air you breathe faithfully permeates your body, the spirit of life energy is flowing through you now.

Whether you pray five times a day while facing east or you only pray on Easter, whether it's regimented or only when you get into trouble, the point is it's all centered around *faith;* A faith in something that is larger than us that has the ability to work in our lives. We may not fully understand, but we can believe and have faith it works.

As you pursue a healthy physical life through conscious breathing, sufficient hydration, pure whole nutrition, fun movement, enjoyable sex and deep, regenerative rest, I encourage you to also achieve the richness and fulfillment of a healthy spiritual life.

REVIEW: ESSENTIALS

1. **Oxygen:** Do your cleansing breath exercises.
2. **Water:** Drink half your weight in ounces throughout the day or simply keep your urine clear.
3. **Food:** Eat 70% living raw foods, and be tested for food toxicity and hormonal imbalances.
4. **Movement:** Do at least 30 minutes of fun aerobic activity daily and add movement to everything you do.
5. **Sex:** Do it often and make it enjoyable.
6. **Rest:** Get up and go to bed at the same time in a clean, uncluttered environment.
7. **Spirituality:** Set aside time for meditation, prayer, or some type of spiritual practice and connect with your life energy.

Before you move on to the next level, answer the following questions:

1. Did you put into ACTION the one thing that you committed to from the previous chapter? *If not, get your move on! Go back and review the chapter, and commit!*
2. What was the MOST VALUABLE THING that you gained from this chapter?*
3. What is the ONE THING that you can put into action TODAY?*

* Turn to **Chapter 8: Mastering Vitality Simple Plan** and write your answers in the area provided for you (or write in your journal, on note sheet in your smart phone or any piece of paper – whatever works for you). This is the foundation for building your simple plan.

Chapter 5

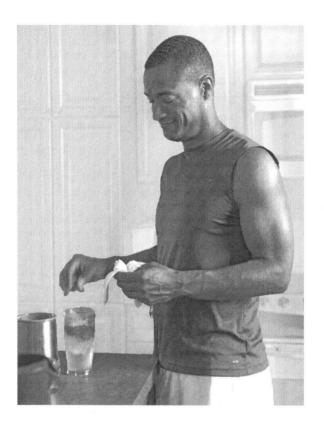

RITUALS

STEP 5 of 7 Steps to Mastering Vitality

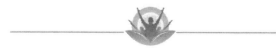

You are a product of your habits, and what you do occasionally matters a lot less than what you do on a regular basis. Your daily rituals create your habits, whether good or bad, which create your life.

You can usually take one look at a person and pretty much tell what their rituals are. If you notice someone who is very fit with little body fat and a lot of muscles, you can assume this person has a set of rituals that include eating a clean diet or going to the gym. Likewise, when you see someone who is morbidly obese, you might conclude that he or she has an inactive style of living and poor eating habits.

If you would like to test this further, sit outside of a Whole Foods Market for about 15 minutes and take a look at the people going in and out. Notice their fitness levels, energy levels and skin complexions. Now do the same for any fast food restaurant or convenient restaurant chain. Do you see that there is an obvious difference in their daily rituals and habits?

RITUALS WITH PURPOSE

Every dentist will tell you to brush your teeth after every meal. Since toothpaste can taste good, you might get a child to do this in order for them to develop a habit of brushing their teeth. However, as the child grows up and if they learn that brushing after every meal leads to bright healthy teeth and less painful visits to the dentist, then the intention of brushing teeth has changed. Instead of brushing for the taste, the child will brush for the long-term benefits.

A habit (like brushing your teeth) is something that is done repeatedly for the sake of doing the action itself. A ritual (like brushing your teeth for the long-term benefits) is the intention of creating a habit by repeatedly doing something with a purpose outside of the action itself.

How much thought do you put into developing your rituals? For most people, it is not a lot. We have a tendency to give ourselves instant gratification by doing things such as drinking coffee, brainlessly snacking or watching hours of television. It is not planned. It is reactionary. You probably don't wake up and say, "Today I am going to drink three cups of coffee, eat five pounds of processed foods, then watch two or three hours of TV while drinking four beers." No!

If you don't plan your life, then your life plans you!

Doing rituals with purpose means that you have the foresight to plan your day in a way that supports the life you desire. Making your plan will be discussed further in the next chapter. What is important for you to know now is that in order for you to make your plan work, you must have the right rituals.

EMPOWERING LANGUAGE

What do you think about in the mornings? Do you wake up thinking about what you have to do? Are you thinking about things that are stressful? Perhaps you rush off to work because you think you need to be there by a certain time. The difference between having a good day and having a day that is filled with stress begins with the words you choose and the meanings you attach to those words.

Want vs. Need

As a fellow high achiever, I am always thinking about what I want to get accomplished. I would also wake up and my first thought would be, "What do I *need* to do today?" This would literally cause my day to start with a false sense of urgency. When you use the word *need*, you are implying that you are required to do something or else you are going to die. You *need* oxygen. You *need* water. You *need* to stop bleeding if you've been cut. Those are things that you absolutely need. Everything else is about what you want.

Reframe

Have you ever said something like this, "I just worked out and it killed me"? Stop right there. Did it really kill you? Are you really dead? No! So, get rid of that language. The first thing you want to do is reframe your language and make sure that it is accurate. This way, you are not telling yourself something that your body, mind and spirit hears. You want to be sure that you are not telling yourself something that is will place limits on you.

If you find yourself making disempowering statements, immediately reframe them. Say, "STOP!" Then ask yourself two questions, "What was it REALLY?" and "What is GREAT about it?"

What Was It Really? In this case, you worked your body and your body got tired. Your workout may have been challenging. You may have been trying something new and it got your attention.

What Was GREAT About It? Well, challenging is good. This way you build your muscles and strengthen your body. You identified something that can give you major gain. You showed up. You actually did the work out. You made progress!

The words and phrases that you use determine the quality of your life. Words create emotions. Emotions create actions. Actions create results. Choose words that create the results you *really* want.

Gratitude

Along with creating a ritual of using empowering language, ask questions that will put you in a state of gratitude such as, "What do I love about my life? What am I excited about? Who loves me? Who do I love?" (These are just a few of the questions that I literally have posted in my shower!) Being grateful boosts well-being. A daily ritual of focusing on all that you are thankful for is linked to having a positive outlook on life.

INCANTATIONS

Another part of my morning ritual is doing incantations. Incantations are something that you say, over and over again, *with emotion*, about something you want to bring into your life. Don't just speak them, *do* them by empowering them with emotion. Some of the incantations that I do while I am doing some type of fun aerobic activity are, "Every cell in my body is grateful," "Every cell in my body is perfectly aligned," "Every cell in my body is connected to the universe," "Every cell in my body is hydrated," "Every cell in my body feels great!"

The key is to do your incantations with emotion. If you say, "I am the master of vitality," power it up by saying it with passion and *be* the Master of Vitality! Use your Power Personality. Breathe deeply, move your body and own it as you announce it to the world, *"I AM THE MASTER OF VITALITY!"* I know this may sound a little crazy, but trust me it works! Remember boxing champion, Muhammad Ali? He was known for his incantation, "I am the greatest!" In fact, he confirmed it by saying, "I am the greatest, I said that even before I knew I was."

After saying incantations over and over again (with emotion), your brain believes it, and then your body aligns to the messages it is receiving. What we think and what we believe becomes our reality, not just mentally, but also physically. You can literally change your body with words and phrases you habitually use.

Some people may think that incantations may be a bit weird or are motivational mumbo jumbo. Yet, we are all doing incantations already. For example, whenever something happens that we don't like, we might say, "Oh my gawd, I can't believe this is happening" or "How can I be so stupid!" What happens is we are charging these statements with emotion. Another example is something we might say in support of our favorite football team such as, "We're number one" or "This year we're going all the way!" This creates a sense of certainty, pride, and accomplishment even though we are not the ones on the field running the ball. Then there are many incantations that we do when we are hungry. For example, "I'm starving" or "I'm famished!" These are all things we are telling ourselves that are not real. However, it makes us feel like it is real and puts us in a state of believing that it is real. Our bodies do not know the difference.

The point is that there are many incantations you are already doing now that do not necessarily serve your purpose. Instead of doing reactionary incantations, intentionally replace them with incantations that are purposeful. It is helpful to make a list of empowering incantations and post them where you can see and say them every day.

PLAN YOUR RITUALS

Make a plan for your daily rituals. Be purposeful and be sure to include things that you can do to maximize your vitality by maximizing the Seven Essentials.

Our subconscious mind is more than ten times powerful than our conscious mind. Therefore, it is more important to program your subconscious mind than your conscious mind. With that being said, the last thing you want to do before retiring for the evening is look at something negative (i.e. the news, a violent movie, etc.). Your brain does not know the difference between what is real and not real when you are sleeping. That is why when you sometimes wake up, you do not know if you had a dream or if it really happened.

After watching the news at night, I used to have nightmares or wake up feeling stressed or scared. The domino effect was that I would be more stressed and tired throughout the day. Then, I changed my nightly ritual to reading something spiritual or listening to something motivational before I go to bed. I go on YouTube and listen to the likes of Tony Robbins, Les Brown, Wayne Dyer, T.D. Jakes, Jim Rohn, etc. This feeds my brain something positive so that it works and loops over and over again while I am sleeping. The result is a more restful night's sleep and brighter, happier days.

The Key to Healthy Habits

When you set large goals, the only way you can accomplish them is by doing something small every single day. Making a clear, sustainable plan for yourself and setting rituals is the best way to do that. Successful people have successful habits. Wealthy people have wealthy habits. Healthy people have healthy habits. Those habits are formed by repeating daily rituals that are purposeful and intended to create a healthier, happier life. That is the key.

REVIEW: RITUALS

1. Rituals create habits – be purposeful and choose rituals that serve you.
2. Use empowering language and know the difference between what you want and what you need.
3. Do regular incantations daily.
4. Plan your rituals to include the Seven Essentials.

Before you move on to the next level, answer the following questions:

1. Did you put into ACTION the one thing that you committed to from the previous chapter? *If not, BE the MASTER OF VITALITY... Go back and review the chapter, and commit!*
2. What was the MOST VALUABLE THING that you gained from this chapter?*
3. What is the ONE THING that you can put into action TODAY?*

* Turn to **Chapter 8: Mastering Vitality Simple Plan** and write your answers in the area provided for you (or write in your journal, on note sheet in your smart phone or any piece of paper – whatever works for you). This is the foundation for building your simple plan.

NOTE: **It is _IMPORTANT_ that you _TAKE ACTION_ and _GET SUPPORT_.**
Connect immediately with someone like-minded such as an accountability partner,
health coach, or professional mentor. **This is key to your success.** *For additional*
resources, support and a **SPECIAL GIFT** *from* **Dr. King**, *please visit*
MasteringVitalityNow.com

Chapter 6

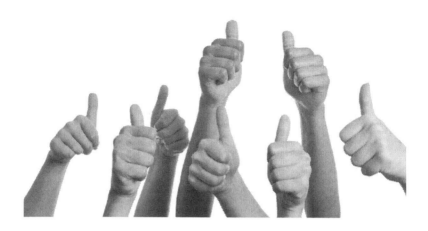

SUSTAINABILITY

STEP 6 of 7 Steps to Mastering Vitality

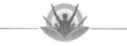

If it were as simple as making a plan for you to follow, we would all be doing that, right? But that's not what usually happens. If you are like most people you make a plan, and then after a while, for whatever reason, you get off track and no longer follow it. What's up with that? Well, I'll tell you. The problem is that your plan is not *sustainable*.

How do you make your plan sustainable? For starters (now pay attention because this is the *most* important key factor in your success), you have got to *make it fun!* That's right. It's that easy – MAKE IT FUN!

MAKE IT FUN!

I have helped lots of people who have had specific health goals, yet they couldn't quite seem to stay focused. They were simply lacking consistency because they were not enjoying the process. All you really need is to have fun while doing at least 30 minutes of fun aerobic movement a day.

Personally, I do not enjoy running for the sake of running. When I played football it was a form of punishment, so as a result, I linked negative thoughts to running. However, you can make things fun if you simply change the meaning you attach to it. For instance, now when I run, I use it as a time to clear my mind and do my incantations. It makes me feel really good. In that way, I have found running to be fun. In addition to, or in lieu of running, I do other things that I love such as Cross Fit, Zumba, basketball, tennis, bicycling, etc. Mary did not like going to the gym, so she took up salsa dancing and Zumba. Not only was she burning about 350 calories an hour, but her social life also expanded in a fun, enjoyable way.

The point is that you need to find out what it is you like to do, focus on that, and HAVE FUN!

SET YOURSELF UP TO WIN

Build on Your Past Successes.

My guess is that there was a time you were at your ideal body weight, you felt energetic, or that you set a goal and accomplished it. You did this because you were meeting certain needs. We all have many needs in life, including the need to have fun while feeling energetic and alive. So ask yourself, "How can I meet my needs?" If you design a plan that satisfies you, then you have a built-in reason for that plan to be successful. Instead of thinking about what you must to do to exercise, think about how you can do a fun aerobic activity that you enjoy while it meets a multitude of your needs.

Ask Winning Questions.

Do not ask yourself questions that predispose you to failing, like "Why is this so hard for me?" Instead, ask questions that set you up to win such as, "How can I do this *and* have fun", or "What is the best way for me to do this?"

Control Your Environment.

Set your environment up so that it helps you to win as well. If you intend to lose weight, get rid of all that junk food in your cupboards and refrigerator! Get rid of temptations – i.e. out of sight, out of mind. Stock your kitchen full of healthy, nutritional foods so that you have them easily on hand. If you need to get up at the same time every day, move that alarm clock away from where you can roll over and hit the snooze button. Put it where you have to get out of the bed in order to turn it off. If you need to increase the amount of water you drink daily, keep water within reach everywhere you go, in your car, at your desk, in every room, etc. Tell those around you what you are doing to master your vitality and ask them for their support. Be creative and think of anything you can do that will alter your environment to your benefit.

RESET YOUR THERMOSTAT

Before you can reach any destination, you have to plan your journey. You will need a roadmap. Once you make this plan, you will then want to stick to it. This is where most of us fall short. It's not that we don't know what to do – it's that we don't do what we know we need to do! Therefore, we don't stay on course. Another reason is because our "Why" is not big enough. We allow old habits to get in the way. More importantly, it is because we have not changed our standards. You set your goals, but did you reset what your standards needed to be in order to get there?

What you need to do is reset your thermostat. What does that mean? Figuratively speaking, it is just like setting the thermostat in your house. If it is too cold, you reset your thermostat to a higher temperature. Your heater then turns on and your house starts to warm up. Eventually, the air reaches your comfort zone (or the temperature in which you set). Once that happens, the heater automatically turns back off.

So, what does this have to do with your health? Let us use weight as an example. Say your *ideal* body weight is 140 pounds, but right now, you hover between 180 and 200. I ask you, what is your weight thermostat set at? Where are you comfortable? The answer is not 140 pounds – it is probably closer to 190. That is why you weigh close to 200 pounds.

When you get to a weight over190 pounds, the thermostat in your brain kicks in and you do whatever it takes to get under that number, or back to your comfort zone. You don't realize that your thermostat is trying to get you down to 190 pounds. You think, because your ideal weight is 140 pounds, that it's trying to get you down to that. But what happens is, when you get down to 185 pounds or so, you relax a bit. You become comfortable and you feel that you can maybe cheat, work out less, skip some weeks in the gym, etc. When you get back up to 195 pounds again, your weight thermostat kicks in and the cycle starts over. What you need to do is reset your thermostat to your *ideal* body weight 140 pounds... then make it a *must* to maintain it.

Now go back to getting leverage on yourself. Making something a *must* is linked to knowing what your "Why" is. Why *must* you maintain your ideal weight? Ask yourself questions such as, "What is it costing me not to be at my ideal weight? Who is it hurting? What am I giving up? Who could benefit if I were able to get down to my ideal body weight? Who will I be when I can move the way I want?" Do you remember a time when you were fit, healthy, active and at a great weight? Even if you have to go back as far as when you were a child, what did that feel like?

That is the standard to set for yourself now. You *can* be that person again. It is alive in you as your Power Personality. Give that personality a nickname and call on it. Get really clear on what it is you want to be, and what standards you are going to hold for yourself. *Then make it a must!*

MAKE A PLAN

Have Your Foundation in Place

Let's first review what you have learned thus far in the **7 Steps Simple & Sustainable Steps to Mastering Vitality**. This is to ensure that you will fully empower yourself. If you are not in alignment with any of these steps, then I suggest you go back and review them until you feel that you are. Trust me, having this foundation in place is key to making your plan successful.

Step 1: CLARITY – You are clear on your goals and have taken full responsibility for where you are right now, what you want, why you want it, and what it's going to take for you to change. You also have a clear mental picture of what your end result looks like, and you know that you must take action in order to get there. *If not, review Chapter 1 and get more Clarity.*

Step 2: LEVERAGE – You have gained emotional leverage on yourself by knowing your "Why and making it big enough to inspire everything you do. You know how to set yourself up to win by making changes around you and controlling your environment. You also understand your culture and how to respectfully influence it so that you can tweak it to your advantage as well as for the good of others. *If not, review Chapter 2 to gain more Leverage.*

Step 3: POWER PERSONALITY – You have found your Power

Personality, given it a name, and now call upon it whenever you want to step up and accomplish anything you desire. You know how to use your Power Personality and be a Vitality Master in every aspect of your life. *If not, review Chapter 3 to find your Power Personality.*

Step 4: ESSENTIALS – You are now aware of the seven essentials necessary for living a life of true health and vitality. You know now to properly breathe, stay hydrated, eat living foods, energize with movement, stay well rested, enjoy sex, and connect spiritually. *If not, review Chapter 4 and review the seven Essentials.*

Step 5: RITUALS – You know that you are a product of the habits that you have created for yourself, and you know how to create healthy habits by doing daily rituals that are purposeful and intended to create the life that you desire. You strengthened your daily rituals by using incantations and positive language. *If not, review Chapter 5 and create your Rituals.*

Step 6: SUSTAINABILITY – YOU MAKE IT FUN, right? Yes! In addition, you set yourself up to win by building on your past successes and controlling your environment. You have reset your thermostat to a better standard and now you are primed and ready to make a plan for yourself. You have reviewed the chapters necessary to ensure that you have it. *If not, review the chapters necessary to ensure that you have it!* If so, read on…

CONGRATULATIONS! Everything you have done so far is why you are well on your way to having a plan in place that is simple, sustainable, *and* successful. Now it is time to write your plan.

WRITING YOUR PLAN

Your Formula for Simple & Sustainable Success

Many people say that they want to lose weight. That alone will not work. You need to write a plan. In order for a plan to work, it must be stated with a non-negotiable intention ("I will" as opposed to "I want to" or "I hope to") and that plan must have each of the following parts:

- **Title** – Name the precise goal in which you want to accomplish.
- **Task** – State what it is you need to do in order to make that happen.
- **Time** – State the duration and time-frame or your task.

Example of a Simple Plan: I will *(intention)* lose 30 pounds of weight *(title)* by doing fun aerobic activities *(task)* at least 30 minutes a day, 5 days a week *(time)*.

For more examples, see Bob and Mary's Simple Plans in Appendix B.

Set Clear and Concise Goals. Make sure that your "Why" is big enough to fully support your plan. Lift the elephant, so to speak. (Remember the million dollars and the gun?) Determine a timeline in which you expect things to happen.

Write Out Your Plan and Post It Where You Can See It Every Day. If it is in front of your view, it is in front of your mind. Seeing and reading your plan daily tells your brain what it needs to do. Your brain is then on alert to seek out opportunities and circumstances that will support you.

Put Your Stake in the Ground

Set Your Goal and Be Flexible. Think of making your plan and setting your goals like putting a stake in the ground with a line tied between you and the stake. The stake is unwavering, that is your goal. You, on the other hand, are on the other end of the line. As you pull yourself closer and closer to the stake, you can move about, tweaking your steps as needed along the way. Things will come up and you will need to adjust. Remember to keep your sights on your goal and keep moving yourself towards it. It is better to tweak and readjust than it is to give up.

Be Kind to Yourself and Enjoy the Process. If you are too hard on yourself, you will most likely want to stop and go back to your old ways. Be as patient and nurturing with yourself as you would with a small child learning something for the first time – and remember to *make it fun!*

Start Slow and Set Yourself Up to Win. It is important to keep reinforcing your foundational base and following through (i.e. doing each of the 7 Steps to Mastering Vitality). If you consistently do these things, you will have a plan that is sustainable. But wait, there's more!

ACCOUNTABLITY

Get an Accountability Partner

No Man is an Island. I have an accountability partner who I check-in with every day. It does not take long; I just shoot him a text. Whenever I have completed my daily rituals, I let my accountability partner know by texting, "Done." He does the same. By doing this, we reinforce the sustainability of our actions and goals.

Do The 21–Day Challenge

Game On! It takes about 60 days or so to create a habit. However, that many days can be daunting, so break it up into three sets of 21–day challenges. Having an accountability partner to do this with you is key. The way this works is you commit to doing a daily ritual for 21 days in a row while holding each other accountable for getting it done. If either one of you misses a day, then you both have to start back at zero. This helps you to be accountable to your goals because neither of you will want to be the one who makes the other person have to restart the count.

There would be times when my accountability partner and I would literally be on day15, and for some reason or another, I would get caught up in the day. It would be getting late, around 11:30 at night. I would be tired and not wanting to do the daily ritual. If it were just me, I would most likely let myself off the hook and not get it done. However, because I knew that it was going to affect him as well, I would push myself. That is what having an accountability partner does, and that is the power of doing a 21–day challenge.

A good friend of mine in the entertainment industry, Havilah Malone, public speaker, and best selling author of *How to Become a Publicity Magnet,* started the *21 To Win Challenge* at www.facebook.com/groups/21ToWin. This group is for people just like you who are committed to making sustainable changes. This is also a good place for you to connect with accountability partners.

Tell The World!

Let Your Intentions Be Known. The more people you tell, the more support you will rally around your goals. Then, not only will you want to do this for yourself, but also you will want to spare the embarrassment of not following through. Being good for your word and saving face are very powerful motivators!

CELEBRATE!

Celebrate and Reward Your Achievements

As you make your plan, be sure to include milestones. This keeps you engaged and adds to the fun. Create rewards and celebrations for each time you achieve something substantial to your progress. For instance, if your goal is to lose 40 pounds, then celebrate for each increment of every 10 pounds that you lose. Make a date for a movie, get a massage, take a trip out of town, go shopping for a new piece of clothing – anything that reinforces your commitment to achieving your ultimate outcome. When you lose your first 10 pounds, celebrate! When you lose 10 more, celebrate! If you wake up feeling good about the fact that you are making any progress at all, celebrate! Heck, celebrate the fact that you are alive! The more you celebrate, the more you release positive chemical substances throughout your body. That in itself is worth celebrating!

REVIEW: SUSTAINABILITY

1. Make it fun! Choose fun aerobic activities that you enjoy!
2. Set yourself up to win! Build on your successes, ask winning questions, and control your environment.
3. Reset your thermostat to your ideal weight, know your Why, and make it a must!
4. Make a plan. Have your foundation in place (i.e. 7 Steps to Mastering Vitality).
5. Write your plan so that your goals state the precise title, time, and tasks.
6. Be flexible and kind with yourself.
7. Get an accountability partner and do 21-Day Challenges.
8. Celebrate!

Before you move on to the next level, answer the following questions:

1. Did you put into ACTION the one thing that you committed to from the previous chapter? *If not, shake your booty! Go back and review the chapter, and commit!*
2. What was the MOST VALUABLE THING that you gained from this chapter?*
3. What is the ONE THING that you can put into action TODAY?*

* Turn to **Chapter 8: Mastering Vitality Simple Plan** and write your answers in the area provided for you (or write in your journal, on note sheet in your smart phone or any piece of paper – whatever works for you). This is the foundation for building your simple plan.

NOTE: *It is <u>IMPORTANT</u> that you <u>TAKE ACTION</u> and <u>GET SUPPORT</u>.*
Connect immediately with someone like-minded such as an accountability partner, health coach, or professional mentor. **This is key to your success.** *For additional resources, support and a **SPECIAL GIFT** from **Dr. King**, please visit MasteringVitalityNow.com*

Linell King, M.D.

Chapter 7

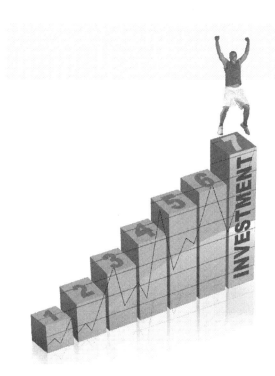

INVESTMENT

STEP 7 of 7 Steps to Mastering Vitality

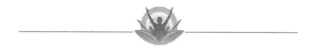

It is said that people who pay, pay attention. It is important to invest your time, energy, and resources so that you can obtain what you really want. In other words, fully invest in yourself in every way, including mentally, emotionally, and financially, in order to fully grow in the direction that you choose for yourself.

Invest Your Time & Energy

We all have the same amount of time in a day… 24 hours. How you choose to spend your time and energy during those hours determines the quality of your life, especially your health and relationships. Unfortunately, too many people are living their lives at a fast pace, trying to accomplish too much and not allowing enough time for their health. The fact is you don't have to create more time. You can, however, utilize the time you already have more effectively.

Mary learned this the hard way. She was constantly placing herself under pressure to work harder and do more, yet didn't take the time to relax or enjoy herself. She paid the price with her health. Not only was she steadily gaining weight, but she was also battling insomnia, fatigue, aches and pains, and frequent headaches. One day, Mary noticed a lump in her right breast. Since she had a history of cancer in her family (and the fact that she was post menopausal), Mary became immediately alarmed and made an appointment right away.

Mary had not believed that she had the time or energy to take care of her health, yet she found herself being forced to use both in order to deal with the possibility of cancer. In addition, the extra worry and stress she experienced while waiting for the test results kept her from concentrating on anything else. It was most disruptive to her life as she literally came face-to-face with her own mortality.

Fortunately, the biopsy showed the lump to be benign (not cancerous). While this was a huge relief, Mary knew that she had been playing roulette with her health and this scare forced her to make a change before it was too late.

By taking the time to write out a simple plan, you will actually save yourself more time and energy in the long run. In Mary's case, once she had a plan and started making healthier choices, her energy and vitality increased tenfold. She was then able to think more clearly, run her life more efficiently and actually enjoy some free time.

Invest in Yourself Mentally

Get your mind invested mentally by *knowing* the consequences of your actions. Know what will happen if you *don't* make the change. Once Mary got the wake-up call, she was able to wrap her head around the fact that she was solely responsible for her actions. Be fully aware of how desperately you hurt yourself as well as those you care for when you *don't* take care of yourself. Think about your rewards. Keep these thoughts in the forefront of your mind.

Once you have your plan written, be sure to stay focused on it. Carry it around with you, keep it on your smart phone or post it where you can see it every day. As discussed in Steps 1 and 2, get into the right state of mind by being absolutely clear on where you are; know exactly what you want for yourself and why you want it. Investing in yourself mentally with this type of clarity and leverage is important.

Get Emotionally Invested

To invest yourself emotionally, not only do you need to know the consequences of your actions, but you also must deeply *feel* consequences of your outcomes. Let yourself feel the truth of what is happening in your life. Emotionalize your "Why" and let nothing stop you. Continually revisit Step 2 and gain emotional leverage on yourself. The more you invest emotionally, the more charge you can add to your momentum, which leads to quicker, more sustainable results.

As you read further, go through and actually visualize your answers to the following questions. Do not just read them – go deep and become connected with what you truly and genuinely want for yourself:

- If you could have your health and vitality *exactly* how you wanted it (as if you could paint your perfect picture of it), what would it be? Feel it. What would be the best part about it? *Why* would that be the best part about it?

- Of those you care about, who would be most influenced in a positive way by you being in your best health and vitality? Who do you love and who loves you the most?
- Who are the people in your life that you would be able to help?
- How would being in your ultimate health and vitality improve your career? Imagine it. How would this affect your finances?
- What would your life be like five and ten years from now if your health and vitality was *exactly* how you wanted it? What would be the best part about it? *Why* would that be the best part about it?

Invest in Yourself Financially

The most effective investment you can make in yourself is financially. Think about it. When you have successfully seen things all the way through to the end, it is usually because you have backed it up with a significant financial investment. College is one of them. For example, just my Medical School loans took me 20 years to pay off. After making an investment of that size, I felt that I had no choice but to follow through!

If you were to review the business opportunities that you have persevered through all the challenges, most likely you would find that they were the ones where you had a sizable investment. If your investment were small, then you would think nothing of moving onto the next thing. So, invest in yourself on every level, especially financially.

Most importantly, invest in your health and do whatever it takes to *prevent* illnesses and diseases. People want the insurance companies to pay for their healthcare, but that is like drinking a poison then hoping someone else will pay for the antidote. Unfortunately, this is the society that we live in and it reflects how we are treating our healthcare. As I mentioned earlier, people invest more in their cars than they do their bodies. It is imperative to make that same investment in your body and get on a steady diet of healthy living foods. The standard American diet (also known as SAD) is making our society fat and sick. The factory farm and food industries are more than happy to take your money. Do your health a favor… take control and invest in the right foods.

I understand it is not easy to do this on your own, nor do I recommend it. There are many things that you can do now and several resources readily available to you. Connect with a health coach or professional mentor. This type of support is invaluable. Get clever and hire a personal shopper to pick up and prepare your foods. Plan your free time and vacations to be in places where health is a priority. Take it to the next level and team up with like-minded people by joining mastermind groups or attending health seminars and retreats. Being a part of peer groups like these not only increases your baseline of healthy lifetime friendships, but also creates a circle of support that catapults you into the life that you desire.

These are just of few of the steps that you can take immediately that will set you apart from the masses. The point is to take action. Invest in yourself to set yourself up to win. It is the smartest investment you will ever make!

REVIEW: INVESTMENT

1. Be willing to invest time and energy to get the life you want.
2. Invest in yourself mentally by knowing your consequences and rewards.
3. Get emotionally invested by going deep and truly connecting with what is real in your life.
4. Invest in yourself financially to reinforce your power and reason for making things happen.

Before you move on to the next level, answer the following questions:

1. Did you put into ACTION the one thing that you committed to from the previous chapter? *If not, invest in yourself now! Go back and review the chapter, and commit!*
2. What was the MOST VALUABLE THING that you gained from this chapter?*
3. What is the ONE THING that you can put into action TODAY?*

* Turn to **Chapter 8: Mastering Vitality Simple Plan** and write your answers in the area provided for you (or write in your journal, on note sheet in your smart phone or any piece of paper – whatever works for you). This is the foundation for building your simple plan.

NOTE: It is _IMPORTANT_ that you _TAKE ACTION_ and _GET SUPPORT_.
*Connect immediately with someone like-minded such as an accountability partner, health coach, or professional mentor. **This is key to your success.** For additional resources, support and a **SPECIAL GIFT** from **Dr. King**, please visit MasteringVitalityNow.com*

Chapter 8

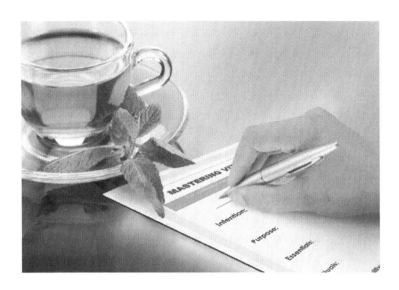

MASTERING VITALITY
SIMPLE PLAN

The Foundation for Building Your Simple Plan

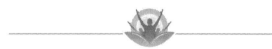

Each of the previous chapters ended with questions for you to write your answers here. If you have not already done so, please take the time now to do so. This is important for getting the results you truly want and the basis for building your Simple Plan is dependent on groundwork you do. Each of the 7 Steps were designed to bring you to this point. Once you have completed this exercise, then move on to the following section and actually write your Simple Plan.

STEP 1: CLARITY

What was the MOST VALUABLE THING that you gained from this chapter?

Your Answer:

What is the ONE THING that you can put into action TODAY to help you get CLAIRITY?

Your Answer:

STEP 2: LEVERAGE

What was the MOST VALUABLE THING that you gained from this chapter?

Your Answer:

What is the ONE THING that you can put into action TODAY to help you gain LEVERAGE?

Your Answer:

STEP 3: POWER PERSONALITY

What was the MOST VALUABLE THING that you gained from this chapter?

Your Answer:

What is the name of your POWER PERSONALITY?

Your Answer:

What is the ONE THING that you can put into action TODAY that helps you live in your POWER PERSONALITY?

Your Answer:

STEP 4: ESSENTIALS

What was the MOST VALUABLE THING that you gained from this chapter?

Your Answer:

What is the ONE THING that you can put into action TODAY to help you incorporate the ESSENTIALS into your daily life?

Your Answer:

STEP 5: RITUALS

What was the MOST VALUABLE THING that you gained from this chapter?

Your Answer:

What is the ONE THING that you can put into action TODAY to incorporate RITUALS into your daily life?

Your Answer:

STEP 6: SUSTAINABLITY

What was the MOST VALUABLE THING that you gained from this chapter?

Your Answer:

What is the ONE THING that you can put into action TODAY to help you make your plan SUSTAINABLE?

Your Answer:

STEP 7: INVESTMENT

What was the MOST VALUABLE THING that you gained from this chapter?

Your Answer:

What is the ONE THING that you can put into action TODAY to mentally, emotionally or financially INVEST in yourself?

Your Answer:

NOW WRITE YOUR SIMPLE PLAN

Most plans fail because people try to do too much at one time. The idea of a Simple Plan is for you to start simple and then build upon it. As you begin mastering one thing, you can then add another.

Write your Simple Plan using the following five easy steps (to see what this looks like, take a look at Bob and Mary's Simple Plans in Appendix B on page 138).

Step 1: Set Your Intention

Using the present tense as if it has already happened, write down what you want to accomplish. Remember, your brain does not know the difference and will comply with whatever you tell it to do. You amplify the power of your statement by stating it using the words, "I am".

For example:

Intention: I am at my ideal weight of 130 pounds and feeling happy, healthy, vibrant, and successful in everything I do.

Now Write Your Intention:

Step 2: Set Your Purpose

Using the leverage you have on yourself, state your reason "Why" you are Mastering your Vitality.

For example:

Purpose: The purpose of Mastering my Vitality is to have energy so that I can play with my grandkids, be a positive role model to those I love, wear the close I desire, and to get my sexy on!

Now Write Your Purpose:

Step 3: Set Your Goals

In the following categories, choose at least ONE THING that you can begin now. You can certainly list more if you wish – just remember to set yourself up to win!

ESSENTIALS: Choose at least one Essential that you will take action now to improve, and then write down next to it at least ONE ACTION you will take in order to get the result you want. Remember to state your intention including title, time and task.

For example:

1) Oxygen
2) Water
3) Food
4) Movement √
5) Rest
6) Sex
7) Spirituality

Movement: I am doing fun aerobic activities at least 30 minutes a day, 5 days a week.

Now Write Your Essential Goal:

RITUALS: Choose at least one Ritual that you will take action now to implement, then write down next to it at least ONE ACTION you will take in order to get the result you want. Remember to use empowering language and charge it with emotion.

For example:

Incantations: Every hour on the hour, I am announcing to the world that EVERY CELL IN MY BODY IS FILLED WITH JOY & VITALITY!

Now Write Your Ritual Goal:

SUSTAINABILITY: Choose at least ONE ACTION you will take now to make your plan Sustainable and then write down what you want the result to look like. Remember to make it fun!

For example:

Accountability: I am committed to my accountability partner and text DONE! after doing my daily incantations.

Now Write Your Sustainability Goal:

INVESTMENT: Choose at least ONE ACTION you will take now to Invest in yourself, and then write down what you want the result to look like. Remember to make your time and energy worthwhile by investing mentally, emotionally and financially.

For example:

Investment: I am showing up and bringing my enthusiasm to the next live Vitality event and connecting with at least three like-minded people as we support each other in reaching our goals.

Now Write Your Sustainability Goal:

Step 4: Power It Up

Use the MASTERING VITALITY: SIMPLE PLAN form (see Appendix C, page 38) or simply get a blank piece of paper. Write your Power Personality name across the top of it and write your Simple Plan below it.

Step 5: Post Your Plan

You did it! Now post your Simple Plan where you can see it then take action on your goals every day. Make this your new life and remember to *MAKE IT FUN!*

NOTE: *It is IMPORTANT that you TAKE ACTION and GET SUPPORT. Connect immediately with someone like-minded such as an accountability partner, health coach, or professional mentor. This is key to your success. For additional resources, support and a SPECIAL GIFT from Dr. King, please visit MasteringVitalityNow.com*

Summary

YOUR PRESCRIPTION FOR MASTERING VITALITY

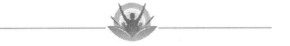

My hope is that you now have a good understanding of the **7 Simple & Sustainable Steps to Mastering Vitality**, your Simple Plan is written and you've posted where you can see it every day. In addition to that, I suggest you keep this book with you so you can refer to it as needed to assist you in staying on track and moving towards your goals.

Your Prescription for Mastering Vitality is to now *decide* and take at least ONE ACTION in order to activate what you have learned.

YOUR NEXT STEP

Decide

You know that in order to get the results you want, you must take action. You *know* what that ONE ACTION is for you. The answer is inside of you right now. Your next step is to make the decision – *decide what that ONE thing is, then take action.*

Ask yourself, "What is the ONE ACTION that I know would propel me forward into the place that I desire to be?" Just one thing, what would that action be?

Take One Action Now

Sometimes, we are so caught up thinking about what we need to do that we can get overwhelmed, and then we don't take any action at all. For me, I knew that I wanted to be surrounded by people who were going in the same direction as me. I wanted to have constant reminders and accountability. I wanted to get into a group of people where the standards were at a level that I dreamed of for myself. I knew that would happen if I went to seminars and live events. I intellectually knew what to do and could even put together a plan for myself, but the one thing that was really going to cause me to act upon that plan was for me to make it real by getting fully committed... all in... no going back... this is my new destiny... my new vision for myself... period. Therefore, my ONE ACTION was to show up. That's it. Just show up.

I showed up to my first event and everything else grew from there. I met an astounding amount of like-minded people and accountability partners who not only helped me to propel forward, but also turned into lifetime friends. All of this led to the connections that have helped to create my programs and radio show – even this book that you are reading now. By taking that ONE ACTION of just showing up, doors of opportunity opened in ways that I could never have imagined!

Know Your Options

What I like about getting involved with programs is that it takes the guesswork out of achieving your goals. They are designed as clear guidance systems set up to ensure your success. They help you save time and frustration, get your goals accomplished quickly, decrease you having to do things yourself and accomplish things more efficiently. I provide webinars, seminars, live events, retreats, and coaching programs that give you more in-depth precision strategies. These are excellent ways to connect with others who give you the encouragement, support, and action plans you need to win.

Like you, I want to be surrounded by winners. Therefore, my programs are not for just anybody. They are for people who believe the follow:

- My health is my most valuable asset.
- I know the value of investing in myself on all levels.
- I am successful in other areas of my life and I am now ready *and determined* to have success in my health, vitality, and ultimately my life.
- I have reached the point where change is necessary *(i.e. enough is enough)* and I am willing to do whatever it takes to achieve my goals.
- I have a positive, winner's attitude.
- I am ready to live a life of Mastering Vitality!

In addition, like you, I do not want to spend time where I am not going to get results. That is why these programs are _not_ for people who are:

- Unwilling to commit.
- Unwilling to invest in what it takes for them to achieve their goals.
- Valuing material objects more than their physical body.
- Expecting programs to work without doing what it takes to make them work.
- Projecting negative energy.

Are You Ready to Pick ONE THING and do it now? YES! Do something that will take you out of your current environment (which is filled with things that trigger unhealthy habits and states). Commit to one thing that brings you one step closer to reaching your goals. For example, a test for food toxicity and hormonal imbalances could be that one thing (contact us if you would like us to send you a kit to get started). Whatever it is you decide to do – ***do it NOW.***

The pathway to Mastering Vitality is a journey. Remember to take it one step at a time and make it fun! Please know that I am fully committed to your success and appreciate the time that you have taken to read this book. You deserve nothing but the best and I hope I have contributed to you achieving it. You were born to thrive and feel alive, healthy, and vibrant. Nothing tastes better than that!

To your health!

Linell King, M.D.

Appendix A

Do You Have Any of These Symptoms?

To see a better view of the Physician Test Indicator Guide and list of symptoms please visit *MasteringVitalityNow.com*

Physician Test Indicator Guide

Immuno Laboratories

"Your success with consistently reliable lab tests since 1978...guaranteed!"

6801 Powerline Road
Fort Lauderdale, FL 33309-2215
Phone: (954) 691-2500
Toll Free: (800) 231-9197
Fax: (954) 691-2505
www.ImmunoLabs.com

Specific combinations of symptoms may be an indicator that additional tests are required in order to rule out underlying chronic health conditions.

Condition-Specific Symptoms associated with food allergies, Candida, Gliadin and IgE

Assays

Food Allergy IgG: 77/87 symptoms listed below indicate a delayed food allergy* — Food Allergy/IgG ●
IgE: 23/87 symptoms listed below indicate an immediate reaction to foods and/or airborne allergens** — Total IgE ◆
Candida: 12/35 Candida symptoms listed below are common to both Food Allergy/IgG and Gliadin*** — Candida ▲
Gliadin: 12/17 symptoms of Gliadin are common to Food Allergy IgG and Candida**** — Anti-Gliadin ■

Digestive Tract		Head		Nose	
Belching	● ▲	Dizziness	● ◆	Excessive mucous	● ◆
Bloated feeling	● ▲ ■	Faintness	●	Hay fever	● ◆
Constipation	● ▲ ■	Headaches	● ■ ◆	Sinus problems	●
Diarrhea	● ▲ ■ ◆	Insomnia	● ▲	Sneezing attacks	● ◆
Nausea	◆	Lightheadedness	◆	Stuffy nose	● ◆
Passing gas	● ▲ ■	**Joint & Muscles**		**Skin**	
Stomach pains	● ▲ ■	Aches in muscles	● ▲ ■	Acne	●
Vomiting	◆	Arthritis	● ▲	Angioedema	◆
Ears		Feeling of weakness	● ▲	Dermatitis	◆
Drainage from ear	●	Limited movement	● ▲	Eczema	◆
Ear aches	●	Pain in joints	● ▲ ■	Excessive sweating	●
Ear infections	●	Stiffness	● ▲	Flushing/hot flashes	●
Hearing loss	●	**Lungs**		Hair loss	●
Itchy ears	● ◆	Asthma, bronchitis	●	Hives, rashes	● ■ ◆
Ringing in ears	●	Chest congestion	●	Itching	◆
Emotions		Difficulty breathing	●	**Weight**	
Aggressiveness	●	Shortness of breath	●	Binge eating	● ▲
Anxiety, fear	● ▲	Wheezing	◆	Compulsive eating	● ▲
Depression	● ▲ ■	**Mind**		Cravings	● ▲
Irritability, anger	● ▲ ■	Confusion	● ▲	Excessive weight	● ▲ ■
Mood swings	● ▲	Learning disabilities	● ▲	Underweight	● ■
Nervousness	● ▲	Poor concentration	● ▲	Water retention	● ▲
Energy & Activity		Poor memory	● ▲	**Other**	
Apathy	● ▲	Stuttering/stammering	● ▲	Anaphylactic reactions	◆
Fatigue	● ▲ ■	**Mouth & Throat**		Chest pains	●
Hyperactivity	● ▲	Canker sores	● ■	Frequent illness	● ▲
Lethargy	● ▲ ■	Chronic coughing	● ◆	Genital itch	● ▲
Restlessness	● ▲	Gagging	●	Irregular heartbeat	●
Sluggishness	●	Laryngeal edema	◆	Rapid heartbeat	●
Eyes		Often clear throat	●	Urgent urination	● ▲
Blurred vision	●	Sticky eyelids	●		
Dark circles	●	Swollen eyelids	●		
Itchy eyes	● ◆	Watery eyes	● ◆		
		Sore throat	●		
		Swollen tongue/lips/gums	● ■		

*See *Immuno Health Guide*, **See *IgE Advantage* brochure, ***See *Is This The Answer To Your Health Problems?* brochure, ****See *Anti-Gliadin Antibody Assay* brochure

© 2008 Immuno Laboratories, Inc.   PCS Doc Physician Test Indicator Guide 121808

Appendix B

SAMPLES OF SIMPLE PLANS

Bob's Simple Plan

Power Personality: BULLDOZER

Intention: *I am at my ideal weight of 180 lbs., my business is successful, and my wife Susie and I are enjoying a passionate relationship filled with love, adventure and excitement.*

Purpose: *My purpose for Mastering my Vitality is so that I can improve my sex life, enhance my relationships, be the best role model for my son and to maximize my energy and take my business to the next level.*

Essentials: *I am power-walking every day for 30 minutes and lifting weights with my personal trainer for 50 minutes every Monday, Wednesday and Friday.*

Rituals: *I start every day with as many push-ups as I can do, juicing 12 ounces of fresh fruits & vegetables and telling my wife how beautiful she is.*

Sustainability: *I am holding myself accountable by doing consecutive 21-Day challenges with two accountability partners. I text to them Done! after I do my power-walking every day.*

Investment: *I have invested in myself by hiring a health coach mentor to keep me on track and accomplishing my weight loss goals.*

Mary's Simple Plan

Power Personality: PRINCESS OF POWER

Intention: *I am maintaining my ideal weight of 115 lbs. and living the life of my dreams of being absolutely healthy, vibrant and energetic!*

Purpose: *My purpose for Mastering my Vitality to be the healthiest, sexiest, most energetic version of myself so that I can inspire other to do the same.*

Essentials: *I am hydrating my body by drinking half my body weight in ounces before 7:00 every night and eating at least 70% organic raw living foods every day.*

Rituals: *I am practicing a morning ritual of stretching and loving my body for at least 20 minutes each day while being in a state of absolute gratitude and peace.*

Sustainability: *I am the Princess of Power leading my accountability partner to victory by texting Done! every day before 11 AM after I do my morning ritual.*

Investment: *I am showing up to a minimum of three Ultimate Vitality live events this year.*

NOTE: *It is* **IMPORTANT** *that you* **TAKE ACTION** *and* **GET SUPPORT**. *Connect immediately with someone like-minded such as an accountability partner, health coach, or professional mentor.* **This is key to your success.** *For additional resources, support and a* **SPECIAL GIFT** *from* **Dr. King**, *please visit MasteringVitalityNow.com*

Appendix C

MASTERING VITALITY: SIMPLE PLAN

For additional support and free resources from Dr. King, please visit
www.MasteringVitalityNow.com

(Your Power Personality Name)

Intention:

Purpose:

Essentials:

Rituals:

Sustainability:

Investment

About the Author

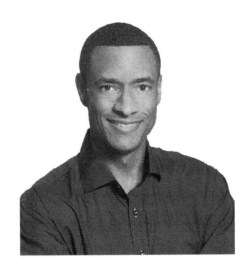

Linell King, M.D.

Dr. Linell King is an internal medicine physician who received his medical degree at the University of Wisconsin School of Medicine in 1997. He completed his residency at The Johns Hopkins University / Sinai Hospital program in Internal Medicine in 2000.

An avid proponent of preventative health and wellness, Dr. King realized the answer to the high incidence of preventable illnesses was to empower the individual to take responsibility for their health. Dr. King published two Los Angeles based wellness magazines and served with the National Center for Health Behavioral Change in Baltimore, Maryland.

Serving as a Hospitalist (a physician who takes care of hospitalized patients) since the year 2000, Dr. King witnessed on a daily basis the destruction that preventable diseases have on our society. After experiencing the fatal effect of theses diseases within his own family, Dr. King embarked on a journey to learn everything he could about preventing disease, health, wellness, and wholeness of the human life.

In 2012, Dr. King did a business and life mastery world tour with Anthony Robbins. While on the spiritual aspect of this journey, Dr. King traveled to Oneness University near Chennai, India, where he gathered with people of all faiths such as Christian, Muslim, Jewish, Hindu, Buddhist as well as non-faiths such as agnostic. *"The more I was exposed to the scientific world and other religions,"* Dr. King shares, *"the more my belief was expanded with other possibilities. In India, we were all connected under one roof, all a part of the same universe. The teachings of Oneness University were not of one belief or about whose faith was right or wrong. The focus was on how to connect with our own individual Divine within our own individual faiths. We all have a personal connection to some sort of higher power. How strong or weak our personal connection is depends on our efforts to connect. As with any friend or loved one, our level of connection depends on our desire to communicate with that friend or loved one. My connection is growing everyday now that I am having daily conversations with my Divine."*

In addition to his speaking engagements, live events and Ultimate Vitality Radio Show, Dr. King works privately with individuals to take their health and vitality to the next level by helping them breakthrough challenges with weight loss and chronic disease.

For more information, visit *MasteringVitalityNow.com* or *MeetDrKing.com*

INDEX

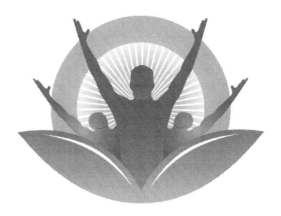

MasteringVitalityNow.com

Made in the USA
Middletown, DE
16 January 2020